Connie W. Bales is Associate Director of the Sarah W. Stedman Center for Nutritional Studies, Associate Professor of Medicine, and Senior Fellow at the Center for the Study of Aging and Human Development at Duke University Medical Center. She holds a doctorate in Nutrition Science and is also a Registered Dietician.

Laura Svetkey is Associate Professor of Medicine and Director of the Hypertension Center at Duke University Medical Center. She is an active member of the faculty at the Stedman Center for Nutritional Studies, where she conducts research on nutritional aspects of high blood pressure.

Pao-Hwa Lin has a doctorate in nutrition and is the Director of the Clinical Nutrition Research Unit at the Stedman Center.

Tamara Shusterman is a Registered Dietician with a master's degree in public health, and conducts research, counsels patients, and teaches nutrition at the Stedman Center.

Dietary Approaches to Healthy Living
from
The Sarah W. Stedman Center
for Nutritional Studies at
Duke University Medical Center

EATING WELL, LIVING WELL
with
HYPERTENSION

Laura P. Svetkey, M.D., M.H.S.
Tamara Shusterman, M.P.H., R.D.
Pao-Hwa Lin, PH.D.

Connie W. Bales, PH.D., R.D.
Series Editor

with Aries Keck

VIKING

VIKING
Published by the Penguin Group
Penguin Books USA Inc., 375 Hudson Street,
New York, New York 10014, U.S.A.
Penguin Books Ltd, 27 Wrights Lane,
London W8 5TZ, England
Penguin Books Australia Ltd, Ringwood,
Victoria, Australia
Penguin Books Canada Ltd, 10 Alcorn Avenue,
Toronto, Ontario, Canada M4V 3B2
Penguin Books (N.Z.) Ltd, 182–190 Wairau Road,
Auckland10, New Zealand

Penguin Books Ltd, Registered Offices:
Harmondsworth, Middlesex, England

First published in 1996 by Viking Penguin,
a division of Penguin Books USA Inc.

10 9 8 7 6 5 4 3 2 1

Publisher's Note
The ideas, procedures, and suggestions contained in this book are not
intended as a substitute for consulting with your physician. All
matters regarding your health require medical supervision.

Library of Congress Cataloging in Publication Data

Svetkey, Laura P.
    Eating well, living well with hypertension / Laura P. Svetkey,
Tamara Shusterman, Pao-Hwa Lin.
        p. cm.
    "Dietary approaches to healthy living from the Sarah W. Stedman
Center for Nutritional Studies at Duke University Medical Center."
    Includes bibliographical references and index.
    ISBN 0-670-86658-X (alk. paper)
    1. Hypertension—Diet therapy.   I. Shusterman, Tamara.   II. Lin,
Pao-Hwa.   III. Duke University.   Sarah W. Stedman Center for
Nutritional Studies.   IV. Title.
RC685.H8S867   1996
616.1′320654—dc20   95–25833

This book is printed on acid-free paper.

⊗

Printed in the United States of America
Set in Minion

Contents

Foreword   *vii*

One
Why Is Diet Important?   1

Two
What Is High Blood Pressure
and What Causes It?   9

Three
What Works—Nutrient by
Nutrient   23

Four
How to Eat Healthily   31

Five
Strategies for Buying,
Cooking, and Enjoying
Eating Healthily   48

Six
Eating Out   60

Seven
Weight Control   68

Eight
Recipes   77

Resources and Further Reading   *144*
Index   *145*

Foreword

Good nutrition is the cornerstone of good health. At the Sarah W. Stedman Center for Nutritional Studies, we are committed to the idea that optimum health care includes comprehensive nutritional care. At the Nutrition Center, we routinely incorporate the results of research studies on nutrition and disease into the medical/health care plans of our patients.

The purpose of the *Eating Well, Living Well* series is to share the expert knowledge of the medical doctors and nutritionists who work within the Duke Medical Center community at the level of nutritional therapy and lifestyle intervention. Education is the key to the prevention and treatment of many common diseases. Yet, much of the information available today about nutrition and diet is incomplete and/or inaccurate. We hope that the *Eating Well, Living Well* series will begin to resolve some of the controversies associated with present-day diets.

Many popularly promoted diets are not founded on sound nutritional principles and common sense. Such diets are difficult for most people to follow, usually because there is no consideration for those with special health concerns. That is why we include in each book sections on selecting the right foods in a variety of settings, including grocery stores, restaurants, and recreational events. Another problem with catch-all and fad diets is that there are often no special considerations for individual differences in activity, age, or lifestyle.

The *Eating Well, Living Well* book series addresses these issues directly. We have asked experts from specific fields of clinical research and practice to write about disease prevention by nutritional means, with specific emphasis on individual differences and exceptions to the rules. Each book is uniquely tailored for each disease. This book explores the latest nutritional aspects of hypertension, a disease resulting from increased pressure in the blood vessels that long-term can lead to damage to sensitive organs of the body.

Sarah White Stedman
September 1995

Chapter One

Why Is Diet Important?

High Blood Pressure—The Bad News

I f your blood pressure is 140/90 mm Hg or higher, you're one of the 50 million Americans with high blood pressure. Hypertension is an epidemic in America—nearly one in every four adults has high blood pressure. High blood pressure is the major cause of coronary heart disease, the number one cause of death. It's the major cause of strokes, the third leading cause of death. Every year 2 million more blood pressures creep into the danger zone.

Your body deteriorates from hypertension from the inside out, but unlike the flu or even a heart attack, high blood pressure doesn't cause pain. Yet, creeping within your body, high blood pressure creates havoc through long-term cumulative strain to your organs and tissues. Slowly damaging organs such as your kidneys and heart, hypertension can result in kidney failure, heart disease, and a host of other diseases.

While stress does have some effect on your blood pressure, feeling tense and "hyper" doesn't directly lead to hypertension. The word *hypertension* refers to the increases (hyper) of pressure (tension) within the blood vessels. Hypertension is just another word for high blood pressure, so we (and you) will use both words interchangeably.

The Good News

During the last twenty years, 50 percent fewer people died from coronary heart disease and 57 percent fewer people died from strokes. What miracle drug did these hypertensive people take that saved their lives? The "drug" was a massive education program by the National Institutes of Health (NIH), teaching Americans and their doctors the danger of high blood pressure and the importance of monitoring it.

The National High Blood Pressure Education Program began in 1972 and had immediate results. Between 1973 and 1977 deaths due to strokes dropped by 17 percent and deaths due to heart disease fell by 8 percent. The program taught people to keep track of their blood pressure readings and to treat high blood pressure seriously. Since the 1970s the study of hypertension has been flooded with millions of research dollars. The powerful drugs that were developed have saved many people from the damage and death resulting from high blood pressure.

But taking hypertension medication only keeps blood pressure under control artificially and temporarily. Although taking high blood pressure drugs has saved people from dying of any of the diseases caused by hypertension, people must take medication day after day for the rest of their lives. Scientists are only recently beginning to worry about the effects of drugs, on millions of adults, taken over a long period of time.

Drugs that control high blood pressure do just that—"control" it. You're still one of the 50 million Americans with high blood pressure. While the drugs will lower your blood pressure, their side effects can be quite disturbing because they use many different techniques to artificially lower your blood pressure. For example, some lower the amount of water in your body or block messages to and from your nervous system. Headaches, dizziness, fatigue, impotence, and insomnia are just a few of the most common side effects. Medication can become incredibly expensive. In fact, paying for drugs amounts to roughly 80 percent of the total spending on hypertension. And some of the newest and most effective drugs are up to thirty times more expensive than the earlier drugs.

The same researchers who developed effective drug therapies are now uncovering ways of lowering high blood pressure without drugs. Doctors have found growing evidence that what you eat greatly affects your blood pressure. They've found groups of people whose blood pressures *never* go above normal, and have measured the effects of different diets on groups of people. Scientists believe that you may be able to keep your blood pressure where it is—or even lower it—through nutrition.

The Nutritional Strategy

Nutrition is the *only* way to hold back hypertension's climb without taking more and more drugs. The last twenty years of research on high blood pressure have resulted in strong, direct evidence linking your high blood pressure to both your body weight and what you eat. Changing your diet, possibly even slightly, may result in lowering your blood pressure.

There are two groups of people who have taught scientists that diet affects blood pressure. The first group consists of whole populations in which virtually no one suffered from hypertension at any age. These people, found mainly in remote areas of the world, don't eat the Western diet of highly processed foods, which is exceptionally high in fat and salt and very low in potassium. And the second group consists of American vegetarians, whose blood pressure is markedly lower than the national average.

In 1986 a massive international study called Intersalt began to compare blood pressures and diet from fifty-two different locations around the world. As data poured in from Argentina to Zimbabwe, direct correlations were found between high blood pressure and five different criteria: 1. high-salt diet, 2. being overweight, 3. drinking heavily, 4. low-potassium diet, and 5. low-calcium diet. People in four remote populations—the Yanomamo and Xingu Indians of Brazil and people living in rural Kenyan and Papua New Guinea villages—had virtually *no* hypertension at any age and had the lowest overall blood pressures of all the other forty-eight locations. Their average systolic blood pressure was 103, much lower than the average 120 garnered from all the other centers, and their average diastolic blood pressure was 63, a hair lower than the rest of the world's 64.

What sets these people apart from the rest of the world? Their diet. The average amount of salt these people ate was exceptionally low. The Yanomamos' sodium intake was almost too low to be measured. In contrast, everyone else around the world eats an average of 9 grams of salt or more a day, and many people eat much, much more.

In contrast to the Yanomamos, another group in the Intersalt study, the people of a remote Kenyan village, were found to have slightly higher blood pressures. Migration to cities in Kenya has resulted in greater contact with the Western/industrial world and, as a result, the Kenyan villagers eat much more salt and much less potassium than the Yanomamos. Correspondingly, there is a 5 percent rate of hypertension in Kenya, compared with 0 to 1 percent for the Yanomamos.

These groups of people studied by Intersalt investigators have other factors in common besides very low blood pressures and diets very low in salt. They all have low–average body weights and drink almost no alcohol. Body weight and alcohol intake have been proved to be strong definite links to high blood pressure, but even after compensating for these factors these people's blood pressures are still especially low. Perhaps more important, not a single person's blood pressure goes up as they grow older.

In contrast, after studying people living in China and Japan, the Intersalt researchers found that they have a diet exceptionally high in salt, and that they also have an exceptionally high rate of hypertension.

There are many other civilizations where the people have almost no hypertension, and *all* of them have a diet exceptionally low in salt compared to the rest of the world. In addition, populations that have diets that are low in potassium and calcium also have high rates of hypertension.

Further evidence that diet affects your blood pressure is found by looking at the blood pressures of vegetarians in America. Overall, vegetarians have significantly lower blood pressures than the rest of the population. (And they're not located in faraway jungles.) Their systolic blood pressures are usually about 5 mm Hg lower than everyone else's. This doesn't seem like a large amount, but this little bit can be quite significant. New research on people with normal blood pressure, high normal blood pressure, and those under treatment for hypertension, shows that even small—5 mm Hg—reductions in blood pressure substantially reduce the number of people suffering from major coronary events.

Why do vegetarians have lower blood pressures? Vegetarians have a much better balanced diet than the normal American diet is. They eat more potassium and less salt; they eat greater amounts of different nutrients, through lots of fruits and vegetables; and they eat much less fat. It is a great control group; because the only difference overall between vegetarians and the rest of the population is their diet *and* their 5 mm Hg lower systolic blood pressure, they show that your diet definitely affects your blood pressure.

All of these studies strongly suggest that what we eat helps determine whether or not we develop high blood pressure. If having a diet high in sodium and alcohol, and low in potassium and calcium, and being overweight increase our risk of developing high blood pressure, it stands to reason that following a diet low in sodium, drinking moderate amounts of alcohol, eating more foods rich in potassium and calcium, and maintaining an ideal body weight will prevent high blood pressure. While *prevention* of high blood pressure is not definitively proved, more research is being done here at Duke's Stedman Nutrition Center and by others. What is definite is that a healthy diet can give you untold benefits.

Small changes in your diet can have big results over time. High blood pressure is cumulative, and as you grow older your blood pressure goes up. It takes years for your blood pressure to rise above normal and become dangerous, and it also takes some time for a healthy diet to affect your blood pressure. But it can happen.

To lower your blood pressure without drugs, the Stedman Nutrition Center recommends:

1. Follow a balanced diet—large amounts of breads and grains, and of fruits and vegetables, small amounts of meat and dairy products, and little to no fats and sweets.
2. Cut back dramatically on the amount of salt in your diet.
3. Eat much more potassium-rich foods.
4. Make sure you eat your full daily requirement of calcium—two to three servings of dairy a day.
5. Keep your weight to within 15 percent of your ideal. (In Chapter 7, you'll learn your ideal weight.)
6. Restrict alcohol to no more than two servings per day. One serving is 1.5 ounces 100-proof whiskey, 5 ounces wine, or 12 ounces beer.

If you follow the number-one recommendation —a balanced diet—all the others will fall into place easily. In the following chapters you will learn how high blood pressure affects your body, how you probably "caught" hypertension in the first place, and some techniques, strategies, and even tasty recipes to help you get your blood pressure down to normal and keep it there.

Chapter Two

What Is High Blood Pressure and What Causes It?

What Is Blood Pressure?

Every time your heart beats it pushes blood through your blood vessels. This force of blood rushing through your blood vessels is your blood pressure. It's what moves "fresh" blood to your tissues and organs and what carries away the "old" blood. As your circulatory system listens and reacts to messages from your body, different systems act to keep your blood pressure under control.

Your heart, a small muscle about the size of your fist, beats about 100,000 times a day, pumping 40,000 gallons of blood along the 60,000 miles of blood vessels that make up your circulatory system. With each beat, blood rushes out of the heart into the aorta, an artery the width of a garden hose. Branching from the aorta, smaller and smaller arteries carry the blood to the rest of your body. The smallest of these branch arteries, arterioles, carry blood to every organ and tissue in your body. Within these tissues, blood moves into the microscopic capillary vessels. There it unloads oxygen and nutrients into the tissues and carries away the carbon dioxide and wastes. Mirroring the arteries, a completely separate system of blood vessels, the veins, channels the "old" blood back to your heart.

While it moves those gallons of blood, your circulatory system monitors what your body is doing and adapts your blood flow to your different actions. Your network of nerves, like telephone lines, transmit messages between the circulation system and the rest of your body. When you walk up a flight of stairs, your nerves tell the tiny muscles surrounding your arteries to narrow, forcing blood quickly to your legs. When you're done eating dinner, the nerves tell the muscles to open your arterioles, letting more blood to your stomach. This responsiveness is called microcirculation.

What Is High Blood Pressure?

With high blood pressure, this microcirculation shuts down. The tiny muscles around your arteries are constantly tight, keeping the arteries all over your body narrow. Under this constant stress, the arteries deteriorate, becoming scarred and hard, otherwise known as "hardening of the arteries." The arteries easily become choked off, depriving your heart, kidneys, and brain of blood.

In the past, high blood pressure was considered an inevitable consequence of growing old. But with recent studies showing how destructive high blood pressure is and how effective medication or a change in lifestyle and diet is in correcting high blood pressure, the National Institutes of Health revamped its definition of hypertension. Instead of using misleading terms—mild, moderate, severe, and very severe—the severity of high blood pressure is now measured in stages. Even the category normal has been divided into normal and high normal. The newer terms clearly show the progressive nature of hypertension.

A few small actions today may save you from all the damage hypertension does to your arteries and organs, and may keep you from having to take antihypertensive drugs later in life. "All stages of hypertension are associated with increased risk of nonfatal and fatal cardiovascular disease, stroke, and kidney disease," says NIH. "The higher the blood pressure, the greater the risk."

How Do I Know If My Blood Pressure Is a Problem for Me?

The only way to know if you have high blood pressure is to have it measured by a health professional. Even people with very severe hypertension feel perfectly fine. This is why hypertension is sometimes called the silent killer—because it usually has no symptoms. So get your blood pressure measured regularly before any damage occurs.

Your blood pressure is actually two pressures; first is the rush of blood with each heartbeat, second is the smaller surge in between heartbeats. The first number is the systolic pressure, read as "over" the second reading, the diastolic pressure.

Blood pressure is measured using a blood pressure cuff and pressure gauge, officially named the sphygmomanometer (s´fig´-mo-man-ahmeter). This cuff, which is wrapped around your arm, is a cloth-covered rubber tube. By squeezing the rubber bulb, we fill this tube with air, tightening it and constricting your arm's blood vessels. Then the air is let out of the cuff slowly. As the cuff loosens its grip on your arm's arteries, the heart is able to push some blood past the cuff. You can tell when this occurs by listening with a stethoscope on the artery below the cuff; the pressure of the cuff at the point you hear this pulse of blood is your first blood pressure reading, the systolic reading. Then more air is let out of the cuff, and eventually the point is reached where the cuff's pressure equals the lowest pressure in between heartbeats. The cuff's pressure at this point is the diastolic reading. Below this pressure, you can no longer hear the blood moving through the arteries with the stethoscope.

It takes training, patience, and a good ear to take someone's blood pressure, but anyone can learn how to do it. It is exceptionally important to take many readings of your blood pressure, especially before you begin taking antihypertensive drugs. Also important is to use the right-size cuff. If your arm is very large, with either fatty tissue or with muscle, a smaller cuff won't squeeze your arm enough to cut off the blood flow in your arteries. Interestingly enough, blood pressure readings should be taken in the right arm, not because of being right- or left-handed, but because the artery supplying your left arm enters at a more pronounced angle than the artery that goes to the right. Because of the sharper angle, the pressure of the blood flowing in your left arm is often slightly lower than the pressure in the right. It's also very important to sit quietly for a few minutes before taking your blood pressure. Even walking into the exam room can make your blood pressure look higher than it really is.

Controlling your hypertension begins with detecting it and requires continually keeping track of its ups and downs. Blood pressure is highly reactive, it can vary wildly from one reading to the next, and goes up significantly even when you're just talking. Don't smoke or drink caffeine in the thirty minutes before having your blood pressure measured; each can cause your blood pressure to rise temporarily.

Blood pressure is so sensitive that the mere action of having it checked can make it go up. So many people have anxiety about doctors, doctors' offices, or getting their blood pressure taken at all that there's a term for it; called *white coat hypertension*, it can result in an incorrect reading of high blood pressure. And it can happen even if you don't *feel* anxious or nervous at all.

The best way to make sure that your blood pressure reading accurately reflects your *true* blood pressure is for you and your doctor to base your *high* or even *normal* blood pressure on many different readings over time.

Classification of Blood Pressures for Adults Age 18 Years and Older

	Systolic	Diastolic
Normal	<130	<85
High Normal	130–139	85–89
STAGE 1 (mild)	140–159	90–99
STAGE 2 (moderate)	160–179	100–109
STAGE 3 (severe)	180–209	110–119
STAGE 4 (very severe)	>210	>120

From the 5th Report of the Joint National Committee on the Detection, Evalutation, and Treatment of High Blood Pressure (JNC-V), NIH, 1993.

High Blood Pressure's Effects on Your Body

Arteriosclerosis
Arteriosclerosis is the medical term for inflexible, scarred, narrow arteries. It takes much more effort for your heart to move the same amount of blood through smaller, tighter arteries. The process is like drinking a milkshake. It takes a tremendous amount of pressure to suck a milkshake through a stiff, narrow cocktail straw, but with a wide, flexible straw the milkshake glides into your mouth. It's the same with your heart—a tremendous amount of pressure is needed to force blood through your narrower and harder arteries.

Heart Disease
The effort of pushing blood through these damaged arteries severely overworks the left side of your heart, the ventricle where the "new" blood is pumped out. To pump harder and create more force, the ventricle's muscle tissue gets thicker, a condition called left ventricular hypertrophy. But the heart's larger, thicker walls make it more difficult for the ventricle to expand and completely fill up with blood. Over time, the extra strain on your heart can cause the heart muscle to weaken, leading to heart failure.

In addition, the hardening of the arteries that supply blood to the heart can cause a sharp pain or pressure in your chest called angina. Angina usually occurs when your heart isn't getting enough oxygen, often while you're exercising or doing another strenuous activity. While painful, angina can be useful because it alerts people to the fact that they have a heart problem. But not everyone gets this warning sign. Silent ischemia is when you don't feel the effects of your arteries narrowing. (Ischemia means having an inadequate amount of blood.)

The most dramatic of all results of cardiovascular disease, a heart attack, happens when part of the heart dies. Heart attacks, also called myocardial infarctions (*Myo* is muscle, *cardio* is heart, and an infarct is an area of tissue death), happen most often when a blood vessel from the heart, already narrowed by arteriosclerosis, is suddenly and completely blocked. The blockage can be a blood clot, a muscle spasm, or a large amount of fatty buildup.

Strokes

Chronic hypertension is the number-one predisposing condition to strokes. Although strokes also result from other conditions, your brain is highly vulnerable to high blood pressure. Stroke is the third most frequent cause of death in the United States, and even more people live through a stroke but become partly disabled.

A stroke occurs when part of your brain suddenly stops receiving enough blood and dies. If a part of the brain that is necessary to keep the body working is affected, a person can die from the stroke. In other instances, the person survives, but will have limitations such as weakness on one side of the body, difficulty speaking, or problems with mental ability.

High blood pressure causes stroke in two ways. One, the arterioles in the brain harden (arteriosclerosis), preventing blood from getting to the brain tissue, similarly as with a heart attack. Two, high blood pressure puts so much strain on the wall of the arterioles inside the brain that they break, bleeding into the brain and depriving it of oxygen-rich blood.

Fortunately, you can prevent strokes by controlling your high blood pressure. Treating hypertension reduces the chance of stroke by 40 percent. And in people over 60, treating hypertension lowers the incidence of stroke by 70 percent. These are excellent reasons for doing whatever you can to keep that blood pressure normal!

Eye Damage

The blood vessels in the back of your eyes are extremely delicate and damage easily. If the blood vessels in your eyes are constantly strained and swollen by high blood pressure, they may burst in a retinal hemorrhage, or the vessels may actually separate from the back of the eye, resulting in a detached retina. The eye is the only place in your body where your doctor can look in and see your blood vessels, making it an important part of a doctor's examination to determine the extent of your high blood pressure. Clearly, keeping high blood pressure under control will protect your vision.

Kidney Failure

Your kidneys control the volume of your blood as it flows through your blood vessels and "clean" it of all types of toxins. Just as in your heart or brain, your kidneys are unable to operate if their flow of blood is slowed or halted. Inactive, they cannot remove the body's toxins. Wastes build up in the blood, eventually poisoning your entire body. All levels of untreated hypertension cause decreased kidney function. End stage renal disease, the last stage of destroyed kidneys, caused by high blood pressure, has gone up every year for the last decade and will probably worsen through the year 2000. Once your kidneys fail, you can survive only with dialysis or a kidney transplant operation. One fourth of all dialysis patients in the United States lost their kidneys to the ravaging effects of hypertension. By controlling hypertension, you'll protect yourself from damage to this very sensitive organ.

Risk Factors for Hypertension

The most important risk factor for hypertension is heredity. If your mother or father is affected, you are at risk to "catch" hypertension. But high blood pressure itself may not be hereditary. What most likely is hereditary is susceptibility—a lower resistance to all of the things that cause high blood pressure. You may be genetically predisposed to be more sensitive to the effects of salt, potassium, calcium, weight gain, alcohol, and stress. All of these factors have been found to contribute to hypertension. Having a genetic or inherited tendency can't *cause* high blood pressure, but it leaves you vulnerable to things that do.

Salt Sensitivity

One reason why high blood pressure runs in families may be an inherited sensitivity to salt. When we eat a lot of salt, our kidneys get rid of it. But in many people the kidneys, otherwise working normally, can't get rid of all the salt. When this happens, extra water stays in your blood to dilute the salt. This leads to extra blood volume, which in turn leads to high pressure in the blood vessels, hence high blood pressure.

Salt sensitivity can occur in anyone, but some groups of people need to pay particularly close attention to the damaging effects of salt. For instance, as many as 70 percent of African Americans with hypertension are also salt-sensitive. Hypertension is exceptionally widespread among all Americans, but for African Americans the problem is epidemic. Hypertension occurs *twice* as often in blacks, develops earlier, and is more severe for African Americans than any other group of people. By the time they are 65, nearly 50 percent of black men and 60 percent of black women have high blood pressure. African Americans *can* protect themselves from this damaging disease just by being aware of their risk and keeping risk factors—and blood pressure—under control.

There is no easy test to see if you are salt-sensitive. The best way to see if your blood pressure is affected by salt is to stop eating sodium completely and see if your blood pressure goes down. As we will see in Chapter 4, the damaging effects of salt can be prevented through changing your diet.

While sodium very likely raises blood pressure, other nutrients—potassium, calcium, and magnesium—may lower blood pressure. There is not yet a definite cause-and-effect known, but we do know that all three certainly affect how blood vessels constrict. In addition, calcium and potassium interact with sodium, possibly protecting the blood vessels from sodium's deleterious effects.

Obesity

Being overweight has a dramatic effect on blood pressure. If your body weight is 20 percent or more above ideal, your risk for having hypertension is *doubled*. Americans tend to put on weight in their thirties and forties. As our weight goes up, so does our blood pressure, and the more pounds we add, the more likely we are to get hypertension. Recent statistics suggest that a staggering 70 percent of American adults are overweight.

It may not be the actual added pounds but the mere action of gaining the weight that makes our blood pressure go up. Even if you are not overweight, the pounds you've added slowly as you grow older may raise your blood pressure.

Being overweight is a health risk, but also the *way* you carry your extra weight has implications for your health. Scientists believe that people who have their extra weight around their abdomen, "apples," are at greater risk for heart disease than "pears," who store their extra fat around their hips and buttocks. This is bad news for men, who tend to carry their excess weight around their stomachs, but good news for women, who tend to carry their excess weight around their hips. This may be why men are more likely to have high blood pressure and heart disease than women.

Although it's not easy, the damaging effects of extra weight on blood pressure can be removed through healthy eating. When you have a balanced diet, you're automatically eating less fat and eating more whole grains, fruits, and vegetables. Quick ways of losing weight are almost always ineffective over the long run. It is safer, healthier, and more fun to *add* things to your diet than to take things away.

Following a healthy diet lets you add good-for-you foods, and never means you have to completely cut something. In Chapter 4 we'll go through many strategies on how to follow a healthy diet.

Inactivity

In 1992 the American Heart Association designated inactivity as one of the top four risk factors for the development of hypertension, heart attack, and stroke. Although it is not directly related to diet, exercise is beneficial to your body in many, many ways. It helps you to lose weight, lowering your blood pressure. When you exercise, your blood vessels open up to allow more blood to flow through, helping to keep them loose and flexible, and shielding them from the hardening effects of hypertension. Exercise helps you lose the extra sodium in your body. It lowers your blood cholesterol, cutting the amount of extra fats running through your bloodstream that can clog your arteries.

Just like a healthy diet, consistent exercise does wonderful things for you. And it need not be a strenuous workout. Just like a healthy diet means eating a wide variety of foods in different quantities, healthy exercising means maintaining overall fitness. Cleaning the house, taking a walk on your lunch hour, playing catch are all exercise programs that you can do every day.

Alcohol

Five percent of the people with hypertension probably have the disease because of alcohol. A number of studies have essentially proved that heavy drinking, more than three drinks a day, causes hypertension. This is a *direct* effect, independent of all the other factors leading to hypertension.

Heavy drinking can also lead to hemorrhagic stroke, a particularly devastating type of stroke: the blood vessels in the brain, weakened by years of hypertension, suddenly burst, flooding the brain with blood and destroying brain tissue.

Ironically, when a heavy drinker suddenly stops drinking, his or her blood pressure will surge upward. This is a temporary effect, and after a few weeks of not drinking, the blood pressure should go down considerably. This sudden surge of high blood pressure is very dangerous, especially for people over age 50. If you do have three or more drinks a day, make sure your doctor is informed and you're under his or her care when you stop. But do stop; the long-term effects of quitting alcohol will save years of your life, and not just by lowering your blood pressure.

Drinking excessive amounts of alcohol also works against therapies for hypertension. All of the positive actions you're taking to normalize your blood pressure—antihypertensive drugs, low-salt/high-potassium diet, exercise, weight loss—are hampered by continued drinking. It may even interact with your antihypertensive drugs. Alcohol is also a nutritional wasteland of empty calories and often leads you to snack on salty and fatty foods, both of which promote high blood pressure.

But there is a glimmer of good news. Regularly drinking less than two drinks a day does not carry a rise in your blood pressure. And, strangely enough, recent studies have shown that moderate drinking of red wine is good for your cardiovascular system. Red wine increases the amount of "good" cholesterol, HDL, in your bloodstream. HDL carries fats out of your blood, reducing arteriosclerosis and your chance of undergoing a stroke. But remember, moderate drinking of alcohol means one to two drinks a day.

By knowing your blood pressure, and treating high normal and high blood pressure, we can stop the damage hypertension does to your heart. It takes a long time for such destructive cumulative damage to occur. This gives you plenty of time to begin taking care of yourself.

Many people with high blood pressure will need medication to control it. Fortunately, there are many choices. It is usually possible to find a medicine that will control your blood pressure without side effects. But we would all rather have normal blood pressure *without* pills. And that's where healthy eating enters the picture. In many cases, a person with high blood pressure can eat right to avoid medications altogether. In others, medicines are absolutely necessary, but healthy eating can make them work better, leading to good blood pressure control with less medicine. In those of us with normal, particularly high normal, blood pressures, who are concerned about developing high blood pressure, healthy eating may keep the blood pressure in the normal range for years to come. So we definitely urge you to follow your doctor's advice about treatment of high blood pressure, and we strongly warn you not to stop any high blood pressure medications without your doctor's consent. And we also recommend that you add healthy eating to your high blood pressure program.

Chapter Three

What Works—
Nutrient by Nutrient

The human body requires about forty different essential nutrients; none is a "quick cure" for hypertension. But many nutrients have been shown to affect your blood pressure, both positively and negatively. Scientists are studying the effects of different nutrients, but it's difficult to develop definite conclusions. The effects of a single nutrient on blood pressure may be too slight to detect. Possibly several nutrients consumed together could lower or raise your blood pressure. Maybe untested or unknown nutrients are affecting our blood pressure.

The Stedman Center recommends a low-salt, high-potassium diet because scientists are beginning to find a strong correlation between sodium and potassium to hypertension. This doesn't rule out the effects of other nutrients, such as the possible effects of magnesium and calcium. But scientists, in studying large groups of people, have found time and time again, a direct relationship between a high-sodium, low-potassium diet and high blood pressure.

Sodium

Sodium, found in extremely high amounts in processed foods and table salt, has been very strongly linked to raising blood pressure levels. It is the first and most extensively studied nutrient that doctors found affecting your blood pressure. Sodium helps your kidneys maintain the amount of blood in your body by attracting water into the blood vessels. Too much sodium, however, is thought to overload your kidneys, making it impossible for them to excrete all the extra sodium. Your blood volume goes overboard, making your heart push harder to move all that excess blood and, as a result, up goes your blood pressure.

Our bodies need only about 500 milligrams of sodium to work properly. Currently the average American adult eats about 3,000 to 5,000 milligrams of sodium a day; most of that is salt added to our food through table salt and preservatives during processing. Some foods are naturally rather high in salt, but it is a minuscule amount compared to the heaps we and food processors add. Americans eat much more salt a day than they need. The government describes a high-sodium diet as one of three lifestyle risk factors for hypertension. *The Duke Stedman Center recommends that you eat an average 2,400 milligrams of sodium a day.*

Many scientists believe that as we age we become more and more sensitive to salt, which may be why blood pressure rises as we grow older. It's possible that as our kidneys grow older they become less efficient at purging the salt from our bodies.

However, not everyone who eats a large amount of salt has high blood pressure, and not everyone who cuts the amount of salt they eat sees a significant drop in their blood pressure. An explanation may be that some people are particularly sensitive to salt. People with salt sensitivity watch their blood pressures rise when they eat salt, while others can eat gallons of salt and their blood pressure will stay exactly the same. If you are African-American, you are likely to be salt sensitive, but it can occur in anyone. Scientists believe that salt sensitivity is a major factor in the development of high blood pressure in many people.

Because salt sensitivity is fairly common in all populations, many people who have cut their salt intake have watched their blood pressure go down.

There is no quick easy test to see if you're sensitive to salt. The only way is to eat less salt and monitor your blood pressure. By following the Stedman guidelines of eating a balanced healthy diet, which is inherently low in salt, most likely your blood pressure will go down. Any drop in blood pressure has a ripple effect—immediately lowering your risk of cardiovascular disease and making it much less likely that your blood pressure will rise as you get older.

As more scientists do more research, more questions will be answered. But for now, experience has shown that cutting the amount of salt that you eat and eating more potassium *will most likely* lower your blood pressure.

Potassium

As people eat more salt, they usually eat less potassium. Potassium is a vital nutrient found in high quantities in beans, nuts, fruits, vegetables, and some animal products such as milk and cheese. Processing food adds sodium as a preservative, but leaches away potassium and other important vitamins and minerals. Like sodium, potassium is an electrolyte that helps regulate the water balance between cells and blood volume. Potassium increases the loss of water and sodium from the body, suppresses the blood pressure–raising hormone of your kidneys and adrenal glands, and directly dilates your arteries.

Surprisingly, some studies show that both sodium and potassium have an effect on strokes *independent* of blood pressure. A high intake of salt may increase the risk of stroke, independent of blood pressure, while an increase in potassium, just the amount found in one full serving of fruit, citrus juice, vegetables, or potatoes, was related to a 40 percent decrease in the incidence of stroke-related deaths. This also appeared to be unrelated to any change in blood pressure.

The therapeutic use of potassium to help people stop taking blood pressure medication was shown in a 1992 study published in the *Journal of the American Medical Association.* Fifty-four patients ate more foods high in potassium for one year and found that "increasing the amount of potassium from natural foods is a feasible and effective measure to reduce anti-hypertensive drug treatments."

The Sodium-Potassium Ratio

Although the suggestion that potassium may lower blood pressure has been popular for at least fifty years, the focus is beginning to move away from strictly looking at the effects of only sodium and only potassium on blood pressure to the possible interactions between the two. Blood pressure may be more closely related to the ratio of sodium to potassium than to either electrolyte by itself. Possibly people who are especially sensitive to salt raising their blood pressure are also especially sensitive to potassium lowering their blood pressure. What is very likely is that the more sodium you eat, the greater is potassium's ability to lower your blood pressure.

The evidence is growing for a link between sodium and potassium to blood pressure, and we believe there's enough evidence to act on. More and more scientists believe that these two nutrients have a large effect on blood pressure. But they're still very undecided on other nutrients.

Magnesium and Calcium

Both magnesium and calcium have been shown to lower blood pressures in some studies. However, other studies show that these nutrients have little to no effect on blood pressure. Ongoing research should clarify this issue.

Magnesium probably contributes to blood pressure regulation by decreasing the constriction of your blood vessels. Scientists have found that lower levels of magnesium correspond to higher blood pressures. However, in some studies, taking magnesium pills didn't lower the people's blood pressure.

It is possible that people need a certain amount of magnesium to guard against high blood pressure, but eating more magnesium than that threshold will not provide "extra" protection. You may have to have a deficit of magnesium to see the benefits from eating supplements. It may also be that magnesium's effect on blood pressure works in combination with other nutrients naturally occurring in foods. There's no definite benefit of eating more magnesium for lowering blood pressure, but it's harmless if eaten in a balanced diet. Fortunately, many high-potassium foods are also rich in magnesium. By adding dark green vegetables, legumes, and whole grains to your diet, you can increase your levels of both potassium and magnesium.

Many studies have found that high-calcium diets correspond with lower blood pressures, especially if individuals also have a high-sodium diet. However, calcium pills do not always lower blood pressure. Recent studies seem to show that calcium supplements lower blood pressure only in salt-sensitive people. It may be that calcium has a preventive action against the deleterious effects of sodium on your blood pressure. Another possibility is that people may need to be deficient in the amount of calcium they eat to see any benefits to their blood pressure from taking supplements. Although scientists are not conclusive about the role of calcium in protecting against high blood pressure, calcium is remarkable for its positive effects on maintaining healthy bones.

Fish Oils

Some studies have shown that omega-3 fatty acids (fish oils) are possibly effective in lowering blood pressures in mildly hypertensive men. Taken as supplements in large doses, omega-3 fatty acids have lowered blood pressure in men with either mild hypertension or normal blood pressures. They also stop your blood from clotting, protecting you from the blood clots that cause most strokes and heart attacks.

We at the Stedman Center don't feel that there is a strong correlation between eating a large amount of fish oils and lowering your blood pressure. In addition, many people have serious side effects when they eat large doses of fish oil supplements. The same effect of fish oil that "thins" your blood, making it resistant to dangerous clots, may go too far and lower your blood volume to the point where your organs cannot receive enough oxygen. Fish oil supplements may also contain concentrated amounts of environmental toxins. Unless you are part of a scientific study and under the very close care of your doctor, do not attempt to lower your blood pressure by taking fish oil supplements.

Instead of your taking a possibly dangerous pill every day, a doctor can make many other changes in your diet that may *safely* lower your blood pressure. A more logical approach to eating omega-3 fatty acids, and one that easily fits into a balanced diet, is to simply replace some of the beef, pork, and chicken you eat with fish. Getting these fatty acids into your body the *natural* way is definitely safe. Fish is also very low-fat, and just two fish meals weekly have been shown to reduce the risk of coronary death. Fish richest in omega-3 fatty acids include salmon, sardines, mackerel, herring, bluefish, whitefish, and halibut, with more modest amounts in rainbow trout, striped bass, shark, and squid.

Fiber

The lower blood pressures found in vegetarians lead some scientists to believe that factors such as a high-fiber diet result in lower blood pressures. But tests on the fiber content of diet have shown that eating or not eating large amounts of fiber has an exceptionally small effect on people's blood pressures. Again, it may be that fiber works in combination with other nutrients on blood pressure and possibly these nutrients are naturally occurring in higher amounts in a vegetarian diet. More clinical studies are under way to test the impact of fiber on blood pressure.

But remember that fiber is wonderful for your general health, an important part of following a healthy diet, an important part of a weight-loss plan, and is particularly effective in combatting cancer.

Chapter Four

How to Eat Healthily

After years of focusing on developing different drugs to "fix" particular diseases, doctors are beginning to realize that a healthy, balanced diet may be a better cure than any pill. Through drug therapies, we've learned to cure or control hundreds of thousands of diseases. Now the diseases that kill Americans are lifestyle diseases, born in part from our inactivity and highly processed diet. Keeping within your ideal weight and eating a balanced diet are the best medicine you can give your body.

A balanced diet will combat your hypertension because it's naturally low in components that are bad for your blood pressure and naturally high in nutrients that may lower your blood pressure. A balanced diet can cut your risk of coronary artery disease and stroke. A balanced diet will make you feel stronger and healthier. The longer you follow a healthy diet, the better your health will become.

But what is a "balanced diet"?

A balanced diet is following the daily servings shown on the food pyramid.

A little different from the four food groups we grew up with—dairy, grains, meats, and fruits/vegetables—the daily food pyramid is a better balance of the foods your body needs every day. The four food groups were off balance—ignoring the importance of fruits, vegetables, and complex carbohydrates such as breads and cereals—and it put far too much emphasis on meat and dairy.

Look over the pyramid. Chances are you could

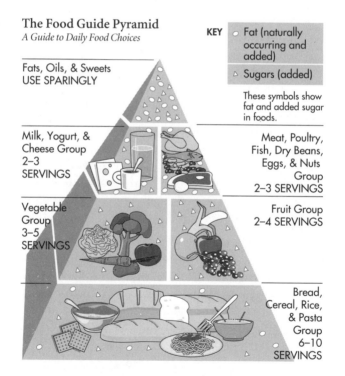

The Food Guide Pyramid
A Guide to Daily Food Choices

KEY ○ Fat (naturally occurring and added)

△ Sugars (added)

These symbols show fat and added sugar in foods.

Fats, Oils, & Sweets
USE SPARINGLY

Milk, Yogurt, & Cheese Group
2–3
SERVINGS

Meat, Poultry, Fish, Dry Beans, Eggs, & Nuts Group
2–3 SERVINGS

Vegetable Group
3–5
SERVINGS

Fruit Group
2–4 SERVINGS

Bread, Cereal, Rice, & Pasta Group
6–10 SERVINGS

be eating *more* food every day by following this healthy guide. When people think of a diet they automatically think of being hungry and deprived. But a balanced diet isn't deprivation; you should never be hungry. And it doesn't mean you can *never* eat potato chips or hamburgers again. The term *diet* is deceptive. We are on a *diet* every day; everything you ate yesterday was your *diet*. You didn't go *off your diet* unless you fasted and ate nothing.

A balanced diet is like a juggling act. If you want to toss in a steak, you're going to have to let go of a few hamburgers. Make changes gradually. Set short-term goals such as "I'll skip a bacon double cheeseburger today so I can eat my favorite lasagna on Friday" or "If I eat three servings of fruit *and* three servings of vegetables every day this week, I'll go out to dinner this weekend." This strategy, of making yourself eat *more* of the foods that are good for you, results in getting you in the habit of eating healthily, with lots of complex carbohydrates, fruits, and vegetables, and with lower fat.

In Chapter 3 you learned what specific nutrients affect your blood pressure. But how do you go about eating or not eating them? *Slowly.* Changing your eating habits is a difficult thing to do. Remember that everything you eat can be "medicine" for your high blood pressure.

Sodium

The key to cutting your sodium intake is to learn to enjoy foods without the masking flavor of salt. The taste for salt is acquired through habit and can be unlearned. Within just two months of cutting down on added salt, your taste buds will actually become more sensitive to sodium. Foods with salt will now probably taste too salty, and you will actually be able to *taste* the food you eat.

The recommended daily amount of sodium is 1,100 to 3,300 milligrams a day. One teaspoon of salt has 2,400 milligrams of sodium, and table salt is only one source of sodium. Sodium lurks in many foods that don't taste salty at all. For example, a half cup of chocolate-flavored instant pudding has 470 milligrams of sodium. Two slices of bacon have 245. One serving of sweet-tasting pudding contains 225 more milligrams of sodium than two slices of bacon. Why?

Processing.

Processing foods for instant cooking involves the introduction of large amounts of sodium, usually in the form of disodium phosphate. The reason for the incredible amount of sodium in the typical American diet is our overwhelming consumption of processed foods. Some unexpected sources of sodium are in quick breads, cakes, and cookies, which use *sodium* bicarbonate in baking powder and baking soda; maraschino cherries, glazed or crystallized fruit, and dried fruit all contain *sodium* sulfite; ice cream usually has *sodium* caseinate and *sodium* alginate as preservatives; sodas contain *sodium* saccharin; and sherbet, jelly, and salad dressing all usually contain *sodium* pectinate.

With all the ways sodium sneaks into your food, how can you possibly cut your sodium intake? Slowly.

A wonderful way to cut the sodium in your diet is to stop buying prepared foods and make your main dishes and snacks from raw ingredients. If you cut down on the amount of processed foods you eat, you can "save" your sodium for when you really want something salty such as potato chips or pickles. Too busy to cook? Everyone is. That's why the grocery shelves and freezers are full of things that will save you time in the kitchen. Prewashed and cut salads, and frozen vegetables already cut and combined into stir-fry or vegetable stew or pasta-vegetable main courses are all wonderful beginnings to meals you make at home. Be sure, however, that you check the amount of sodium. Bookstores are also full of "quick" cookbooks, perfect for you to learn a few quick meals from. In Chapter 8, we've included a few recipes of our own to get you started.

Cutting back the salt you add at the table is also not as difficult as it seems. It just takes a gradual relearning of how food really tastes. In our speeded-up society, too many people choke down food without really relishing its flavor. How many times have you seen people salt their food without even tasting it? Begin to notice how salty many foods taste; after a time you'll want to save your sodium for the foods that you *want* to taste salty. Many spices can enhance the flavor of foods, from pork to potatoes, without salt. Experiment with mints, chives, oregano, mustard, sage; all kinds of flavorful spices will teach your tongue how to really enjoy food again. We've included some seasoning suggestions on pages 52–54. Experiment and have fun—after all you want to eat, savor, and enjoy tasty foods, don't you?

And remember, cutting back on sodium *now*, even if you don't have hypertension, is good for you, your family, your children. It's a wonderful, healthy preventive measure.

Potassium

As people eat more and more processed foods, they eat more sodium and less potassium. Increasing the amount of potassium you eat is fairly simple. Eat more fruits and vegetables. *The Stedman Center recommends that you eat about 3,500 to 4,500 milligrams of potassium a day.* Luckily, eating potassium and having a balanced diet go hand in hand.

Low-Sodium, High-Potassium Foods			
Food	Serving Size	Potassium (mg)	Sodium (mg)
Fruits			
Apricots (dried)	8 halves	490	13
Bananas	1 medium	569	1
Dates	10 medium	648	1
Orange juice	1 cup	496	3
Watermelon	1 slice (about ½ inch)	600	6
Tomatoes, cooked	1 cup	670	26
Tomatoes, fresh	1 cup	400	11
Vegetables			
Broccoli	1 stalk	267	10
Green beans	1 cup	189	5
Mushrooms	4 large	414	15
Potatoes	1 medium	504	2
Spinach	½ cup	291	45
Legumes			
Black beans	1 cup	611	1
Kidney beans	1 cup	713	4
Lentils	1 cup	731	4
Black-eyed peas	1 cup	690	7

Low-Sodium, High-Potassium Foods (cont'd)

Food	Serving Size	Potassium (mg)	Sodium (mg)
Dairy			
Skim milk	1 cup	406	126
1% milk	1 cup	381	123
Yogurt, nonfat	1 cup	579	173
Yogurt, low-fat	1 cup	442	125
Meats and Fish			
Lean round steak	3 ounces	352	54
Lean sirloin	3 ounces	336	57
Salmon	3 ounces	319	56
Scallops	3.5 ounces	393	197
Trout	3 ounces	539	29
Low-sodium tuna (canned in water)	½ cup	323	52

Magnesium and Calcium

Magnesium, another nutrient that may control high blood pressure, is also found in vegetables, especially the green leafy kind. Along with leafy dark green vegetables, whole grains, nuts, dairy products, soy products, and beans are treasure chests of magnesium. *The Stedman Center recommends that you eat a minimum of 300 to 350 milligrams of magnesium a day.* If you follow the recommendation of eating three to five servings of vegetables a day, you can easily get this amount of magnesium in your diet. For example, one cup of cooked spinach and a cup of cooked black-eyed peas will give you about 280 milligrams of magnesium.

Stedman recommends eating about 800 to 1,200 milligrams of calcium a day, both for your blood pressure and your bones. The easiest way to eat more calcium is to eat more dairy products. Dairy products can either be high in fat *or* fat free. For example, one cup of whole milk has eight grams of fat, one cup of skim milk has zero. If you're currently drinking whole milk and skim tastes like white water, go gradually; begin with 2 percent milk and slowly lead to drinking skim.

Cheeses made from skim milk, like mozzarella or other low-fat cheeses, are an excellent way to get in your calcium. But cheese is often very high in sodium. Use it sparingly or as a replacement for animal meats in a meal. Nonfat and low-fat yogurt are both excellent as snacks or meals in their own right, but also as a replacement for sour cream, dressings on salads, or mixed in a blender with berries. (You can eat a serving of fruit and calcium in one tasty shot.) Aside from milk, green leafy vegetables such as kale, broccoli, and turnip greens are high in calcium as is fish with edible bones such as sardines.

Supplements versus Natural Foods

With all our discussion on daily requirements for specific nutrients, you may wonder if the simplest solution is just to take vitamin supplements. A daily multivitamin is fine for filling out the ups and downs of a daily diet. But you *cannot* depend on vitamins to "make up" for an unhealthy diet. Your body needs food, and it's designed to get its nutrients from food, not from a purple-coated pill. Plus there's not much government regulation over dietary supplements. As a result, you can buy supplements that don't contain the ingredients that are claimed, or they may contain contaminants, and it's possible you can take too many and ingest a toxic amount of a particular ingredient.

A major problem of diuretics, commonly prescribed as the first drug to combat hypertension, is they deplete the body of potassium as well as sodium. If you are taking a diuretic to control your blood pressure, you may be losing more potassium than you can possibly eat in one day, and your doctor may prescribe a potassium supplement to keep your levels normal. Following a high-potassium/low-salt diet will probably help combat your hypertension and may let you stop taking the diuretics someday, but speak to your doctor before beginning to take potassium supplements or before you stop taking them.

Fiber

Whether dietary fiber has a direct effect on blood pressure remains to be determined, but its benefits on blood lipids and prevention of cancers are well acknowledged. Also, good sources of dietary fiber are frequently high in potassium. Dietary fiber, found in whole grains, fruits, and vegetables, cannot be broken down by our stomachs. Fiber travels through the "pipes" of our digestive system, acting like a brush and cleaning away accumulated fats and toxins. *The Stedman Center recommends 20 to 35 grams of dietary fiber a day.*

Fiber Content of Foods

Foods	Portion	Fiber (grams
Peas, green	½ cup	5.2
Kidney beans	½ cup	4.5
Apple, with skin	1 small	3.9
Bread, whole wheat	1 slice	2.7
Broccoli	½ cup	2.4
Brown rice, cooked	1 cup	2.4
Apricots, with skin	2 medium	1.5
Lima beans	½ cup	1.4
White rice, cooked	1 cup	0.8
Lettuce	½ cup	0.5

Complex Carbohydrates— the Base of the Pyramid

Your body's major source of energy is carbohydrates, so complex carbohydrates should supply the majority of calories in your diet. They are the base that you'll build upon in making up your food pyramid. Your cells burn carbohydrates, in the digested form of glucose, as the body's main fuel.

Complex carbohydrates, also known as starches, are long chains of simple sugar molecules and fiber. Found in bread, potatoes, cereals, grains, pasta, fruits, and vegetables, complex carbohydrates, like simple carbohydrates, are converted into glucose. But complex carbohydrates are more difficult to digest than sugars so they're slowly absorbed into our bloodstream. Complex carbohydrates are also usually high in fiber, low in fat, and come packed with extra nutrition.

Most of your diet should be complex carbohydrates. *Stedman recommends six to eleven servings of complex carbohydrates a day.* These can include whole grains, brown rice, whole wheat pastas, and breads. More highly processed grains such as white rice and white bread, even if enriched, are complex carbohydrates, but they have much less of what's good for you. There are other grains besides wheat and rice—there's also oatmeal, barley, and corn. Try low-fat tortillas, corn bread, couscous, and kasha.

Carbohydrates probably don't affect your blood pressure, but a diet that's based on complex carbohydrates is likely to be low in fat, and may keep you from getting overweight, which certainly helps prevent hypertension.

Fruits and Vegetables

Everyone has heard the phrase "eat your vegetables, they're good for you." It's very, very true. Research shows that fruits and vegetables are exceptionally important in preventing chronic diseases such as hypertension and cancer. Americans in general consume only three and one-half servings of fruits and vegetables a day.

Eating more fruits and vegetables should be a goal for everyone. Low in fat and sodium, high in potassium, fiber, and other exceptionally important nutrients, fruits and vegetables are an extremely important part of your diet. *The Stedman Center recommends three to five servings of vegetables and two to four servings of fruits every day.*

America's favorite vegetables—iceberg lettuce, tomatoes, onions, carrots, celery, and corn—are some good sources of nutrients and fiber. Unfortunately, leafy dark green vegetables such as spinach, which are so high in potassium, and cruciferous vegetables such as broccoli, cauliflower, and cabbage, which provide wonderful amounts of fiber, are often gravely lacking in our regular diet.

Experiment with other vegetables; you'll probably be surprised with the many different tastes and combinations that exist. For example, iceberg lettuce is only one of hundreds of leafy salad greens. Iceberg, comparatively low in fiber and nutrients, is usually just a tasteless foil for heavy fat-laden dressings. Experiment with Boston or green-leaf lettuces, radicchio, spinach, and other greens in your salads. Prewashed, even pre-cut salads are now sold in ready-to-eat packages. Try them. You'll easily increase your nutrients and need less dressing on these more flavorful leaves.

Also try to experiment with different ways of preparing your favorite vegetables. Try roasting them in the oven at a low temperature, lightly drizzled with a spicy, light olive oil. Try baking and sautéeing them in vegetable broth instead of oil. Try some of the different spices we'll suggest later on. Remember, the goal here is to *eat more!* Now, how often does a diet include *that* instruction?

America's favorite fruit is the banana. High in potassium, bananas are an excellent snack food. But lots of other favorite fruits are also rich in potassium such as apples, watermelons, oranges, cantaloupes, and grapes. A wonderful idea to "sneak" fruits into your diet is to order a fruit plate as an appetizer *before* a meal. Turn a skim milk and berry shake into your afternoon snack instead of eating a candy bar. You'll still get a sweet snack, but with the added benefit of potassium, calcium, and hundreds of other nutrients.

While you're experimenting with foods and

you're moving away from grabbing ready-made frozen dinners, attempt some main dish fruit recipes. Our American version of fruit unfairly limits it to fresh snacks, garnishes, and desserts. We ignore the possibility of fruits as the meal. On a tropical vacation you'd expect meals of different exotic fruits. Why wait? Investigate tropical cookbooks and your supermarket's produce section. Intriguing items such as star fruit, passion fruit, and mangos are waiting for you.

Fruit desserts are another tasty way to consume your two to four servings a day, but, of course, keep an eye on desserts dripping with fat-filled pastry and whipped cream or with heavy sugar glazes. Treats like these are fine—*once in a while.* Save them up, savor them. Most likely, after a week of eating fresh fruits when you sit down to that slice of glazed strawberry cheesecake, you'll realize that you can't *taste* the strawberries under all that sauce; it will taste *heavy.* You *can* successfully change your eating habits; after all it's only a *habit*—not a way of life.

Protein

An important part of every cell in our body is protein. Of the 22 amino acids that build protein, our bodies can make all but ten. Red meat, poultry, fish, eggs, milk, and other animal products are the best sources of protein. Americans usually eat large portions of protein foods—especially animal protein. Animal proteins in general have higher amounts of fat, especially saturated fat. *We recommend that you eat at most six ounces of meat a day.* This is the same size as two decks of cards. Our usual conception, and consumption, of a "serving" is usually much, much more than this. Remember that meat and protein foods are near the top of the pyramid. Instead of being the "star" of a meal, meat should be a supporting actor. For example, chicken stir-fry—lots of rice and vegetables with a light amount of chicken.

Think about the meals you eat each day. Do you feel like you have to eat meat at every breakfast, lunch, and dinner? Replacing meat with "meaty" vegetable dishes will help you reach your goal of three to five servings of vegetables a day and lower the amount of high-fat protein you're eating.

Another excellent way to cut the fat from meat in your diet is to eat more beans, an excellent source of protein, and a way to trade some of your higher-fat meats such as beef or pork for fish. Not only will you cut fat but you'll increase the amount of omega-3 fatty acids, which may lower your blood pressure.

Fats and Sugars

Fat contains the most concentrated amount of calories, and Americans eat far too much fat. The result—the extra fat we eat becomes the extra fat on us. But even if you're not overweight, lots of fat in your diet is unhealthy, especially for your heart and blood vessels.

FAT	9 calories/gram (252 calories per ounce)
CARBOHYDRATES	4 calories/gram (112 calories per ounce)
PROTEIN	4 calories/gram (112 calories per ounce)
ALCOHOL	7 calories/gram (196 calories per ounce)

Like sodium, fat is often "hidden" in our food. While the Stedman Center recommends getting no more than 25 percent of your daily calories from fat, the average American eats more than 34 percent fat calories.

A high-fat diet results in extra fats in your bloodstream. There they build up on the inside of your blood vessels, making your heart pump harder to push blood throughout your body. Combine this with high blood pressure and you're at a greater and greater risk for a heart attack.

The amount of fat you should eat depends on your body size and energy needs. In general, women should have a maximum of 40 to 50 grams of fat every day and men 50 to 65 grams. Although counting fat grams, just like counting calories, is time-consuming and meticulous, it is important to know the amount recommended for a healthy diet and realize that one teaspoon of oil or margarine has approximately 5 grams of fat. That little bag of potato chips you eat without even thinking about them has 10 grams of fat, a quarter of all the fat you should eat every day.

Remember not to weigh yourself down by obsessing on "how many fat grams I've got left." You just want to learn what has how much fat in it and relate that to how much fat you eat every day. It's impossible to follow a perfect diet for the rest of your life. You'll just wear yourself out. Your long-term goal is to eat healthily, enjoy food, and feel better. It is much easier and healthier to lower your intake of fat by *increasing* the amounts of fruits, vegetables, dried beans, whole grain cereals, breads, and pastas you eat. These foods contain significantly less fat *and* fewer calories than their highly processed relatives.

The type of fat you choose is also important for heart disease prevention. Saturated fat, which is solid at room temperature and comes primarily from animal sources, increases blood cholesterol. It should be reduced in your diet. Foods high in saturated fat include butter, chicken skin, shortening, cheese, and animal fat. The type of oils you should choose is monounsaturated—canola, olive, peanut, and avocado oils. Even though one teaspoon of olive oil and one teaspoon of lard have the same amount of fat, 4 to 5 grams, the olive oil is a healthier choice. Remember these oils are still *pure fat* and should be used in small amounts.

Cholesterol is a waxlike substance found only in animal products such as meat, eggs, cream, and cheese. Our bodies make all the cholesterol we need. Too much cholesterol won't raise your blood pressure, but it will harm your heart and blood vessels in other ways. By cutting your total fat intake to less than 25 percent of calories, you're likely to follow the recommendation of eating less than 300 milligrams of cholesterol a day.

While there's been a lot of discussion of "good" or "bad" cholesterol and many arguments on what types of fat are worse for your body (saturated, monounsaturated, polyunsaturated, etc.), it all obscures the basic problem. Americans need to eat less fat.

There's been a boom in fat-free products recently, and Americans have cut their fat intake from 36 percent of their average daily calories to 34 percent. But why then have we gained *eight* pounds per person? One possible reason is that fat-free products just replace fat with sugars that our bodies quickly turn into fat. The flood of low-fat and fat-free products, especially cookies and cakes, is healthier than the originals—*but* these products are not healthier than an apple. And many people eat more of fat-free foods, just making their body convert the sugar into fat instead of eating fat in the first place.

Fat is much more of a health concern than sugar. But for people trying to lose weight, sugar can create a major roadblock. The more sugar you eat, the more you want, and these empty calories aren't beneficial. With the focus turning to nonfat and fat-free foods, many people have forgotten that sugars are also often stored by the body as fat. People tend to eat larger quantities of low-fat foods, especially low-fat desserts such as cookies and frozen yogurt. But they're forgetting that calories as well as fats play a major role in gaining weight. In 1991 Americans ate 164.9 pounds of sugar and other sweeteners per person.

Alcohol

One food category not on the pyramid but important for hypertension is alcoholic beverages. Remember heavy alcohol consumption can increase blood pressure as well as add empty calories and replace nutrient dense foods in your diet. *The Stedman Center recommends no more than two drinks a day.* A drink is a 5-ounce glass of wine, 12 ounces of light beer, or 1.5 ounces of hard liquor.

Chapter Five

Strategies for Buying, Cooking, and Enjoying Eating Healthily

The health tips and ideas that the Stedman Center suggests are not just for people with high blood pressure. Although hypertensive people really need to watch their diet, so does everyone else. We can all benefit from making healthy changes. Don't prepare special meals for the person in the family with hypertension. Don't have a shelf with "Dad's diet food." Your entire family probably needs to eat more complex carbohydrates, fruits, and vegetables. Healthy meals are for the entire family.

Begin by having so many low-fat and low-sodium snacks that they burst out of your kitchen. At the same time, stop automatically buying high-salt, high-fat snacks. If your children or spouse miss and want high-fat and high-sodium snacks, buy smaller quantities. Get one candy bar instead of a bag and bring home smaller bags of potato chips.

The snack packs of cereals and potato chips are good ways to start eating smaller, more healthy quantities of high-fat, high-sodium food. The serving size is already decided, so you can eat the whole bag without polishing off two pounds of chips.

Children and teenagers learn their eating habits at home. More and more research shows that food habits are formed at a young age, which can impact on health problems as you grow older. Remember, getting everyone to eat better takes time and patience. Don't make sudden changes or take an adamant stance. Eating should be fun, enjoyable, not a punishment. Go slowly and both you and your family will be on the way to eating healthily in no time.

Some small, gradual changes toward a healthy diet are:

- Begin buying lower-fat versions of margarine and butter.
- Use spray oil when you sauté instead of liquid oils, butter, or shortening.
- Cut all the fat you use in half.
- Eat two vegetarian dinners a week.
- Switch to types of foods such as mustard instead of mayonnaise, low-salt pretzels instead of potato chips, vanilla wafers instead of Oreos, apple crisp instead of apple pie.
- Limit deep-fried foods and try new recipes that call for broiling and roasting.

In the Supermarket

You'll make your first step into eating healthily at the supermarket. Make a list and stick to it! Shopping after you eat, satisfied with a full stomach, will keep you from grabbing ready-to-eat snack foods and prepared foods that have lots of added salt. Before you throw something into your cart, stop for a moment and decide how it fits into your plan for a healthy meal. All too often we buy products out of habit "because Mom bought it" or "I always buy Oreos." Changing food habits takes time and energy, but remember, you want to *feel better*. Having healthy food available is the first step to a healthy diet.

A new way to approach the supermarket is to shop the perimeter of the store. This keeps you to the fresh produce, bread, meat, and dairy sections. Don't even let yourself go down the candy or snack aisles; out of sight is out of mind.

Begin your shopping in the fresh produce section. The *most important* thing to remember in produce is to *buy a lot*. The key to eating more fruits and vegetables is to have them around all the time; when you reach for a snack, a healthy one should jump into your hand. Buy at least a week's worth of foods high in potassium; you'll find a list of high-potassium–low-sodium foods in Chapter 4. That way, when you want a snack at home or to take with you, things like dried apricots are close by. If you find fresh produce very expensive, compare the prices with frozen vegetables. Quite often they're much cheaper, and frozen fruit and vegetables are still loaded with vitamins and minerals. Experiment with different fruits and vegetables, try some new recipes, and, of course, buy all your favorites.

Now that your cart is full of healthy fruits and vegetables, continue around the store to the breads and pasta. Shop the food pyramid. If you're striving to fill your body with more complex carbohydrates and fruits and vegetables, then make sure your shopping cart is filled with them, too. The bakery usually smells wonderful. Give yourself a feast of whole grain breads and rolls. Try out some new combinations aside from the regular old loaf of white bread, such as darker breads, rolls loaded with chunky grains, and breads topped with oatmeal or barley. Also, try out some of the "new" grains. Couscous is a quick-cooking grain as is barley and oatmeal. In the pasta and rice sections, look for the whole wheat pastas and brown rice. They may be slightly more expensive than the white versions, but weighed against the costs of high blood pressure drugs, hospitalization, and coronary artery surgery they seem quite cheap.

Remember while you're in the bakery section, most cakes, pies, cookies, and unfortunately most muffins (although they look and sound healthy) are loaded with fat. Save them for special occasions. Balance them; don't *make* yourself cut them out. For example, have oatmeal three days a week and then your regular muffins two days a week. You're not going for a diet here—but a healthy way of eating.

In the meat section, remember you need only *two* servings a day. And a serving size is *three* ounces. Save your meat for when you really want to savor and enjoy it.

Try adding more fish. Fish is loaded with omega-3 oils, which may prevent heart disease.

Red meat is the highest source of saturated fat in the American diet, but different cuts of meat vary dramatically in saturated fat calories. For instance, the leanest of the beef cuts is the trimmed, lean, round steak, containing 7 calories of saturated fat per ounce. Compare this to broiled lean ground beef, which contains 25 saturated fat calories per ounce. No one eats one ounce; multiply it by a likely 6-ounce portion, and you get 42 versus 150 saturated fat calories.

Dairy products are a wonderful source of potassium and calcium. But keep your eye on the fat involved. In items where you won't notice the difference, make sure you're choosing nonfat versions. In milk and cheese, choose the low-fat or fat-free options.

The frozen-foods section of the store can be a great place to find quick meals and side dishes. For example, load your freezer up with frozen vegetables. You don't have to cut them up and they can be cooked in a microwave in minutes. Many low-fat frozen meals also work well. Even if the sodium is 400 milligrams, remember you can have approximately 2,400 a day. So 400 is well within a healthy amount. Add a piece of fruit, extra vegetables, and a whole grain roll and you have a quick and easy dinner.

The remainder of the store contains foods that can make your healthy diet interesting and tasty. You may become overwhelmed by the array of different spices. Collect two or three different bottles and try them out at home. Spices are expensive, but one three-dollar bottle usually lasts months.

Suggested Seasonings for Vegetables, Chicken, Meat, and Fish

> ASPARAGUS: dry mustard, lemon juice, marjoram, sesame seeds, thyme, tarragon, vinegar, white, black, or red pepper

BEEF: basil, bay leaves, celery, curry, dillseed, dry mustard, ginger, garlic, green pepper, marjoram, onion, oregano, nutmeg, parsley, black, white, or red pepper, rosemary, sage, savory, tarragon, thyme

BROCCOLI: caraway seed, basil, curry, garlic, lemon juice, oregano, white or black pepper, dry mustard

CORN: green pepper, black, white, or red pepper, tomato, onion

EGGS: basil, curry, dry mustard, green pepper, onion, paprika, garlic, parsley, white, black, or red pepper, tomato, cilantro

FISH: basil, bay leaf, curry, cumin, dry mustard, fennel, garlic, green pepper, lemon juice, mace, marjoram, paprika, parsley, onion, black, white, or red pepper, turmeric, sesame seeds

GREEN BEANS: basil, dillseed, lemon juice, marjoram, mint, nutmeg, onion, oregano, black, white, and red pepper, sage, savory, thyme

LAMB: allspice, basil, curry, garlic, mint, bay leaf, cloves, rosemary, dill, ginger, marjoram, onions, sage, tarragon, parsley

PEAS: basil, dill, lemon, pepper, mint, oregano, onion, parsley, rosemary, sage, savory, thyme

POULTRY: paprika, parsley, sage, thyme, bay leaf, celery, chervil, curry, dillseed, all types of pepper, and peppers

PORK: allspice, apples, basil, mint, vinegar, caraway seed, chili powder, chives, cinnamon, cloves, fennel, garlic, marjoram, nutmeg, onion, oregano, parsley, rosemary, sage, black, white, or red pepper

POTATOES: basil, caraway seed, chives, dillseed,

green pepper, onion, mace, parsley, black, red, or white pepper, rosemary, thyme, vinegar

TOMATOES: allspice, basil, celery, marjoram, onion, pepper, cilantro, sage, thyme

VEAL: apricots, bay leaf, curry, ginger, garlic, lemon juice, marjoram, mint, oregano, onion, parsley, white, black, or red pepper, rosemary, sage, thyme, mace

How to Read a Nutrition Label

As you build awareness of what you're eating, you'll notice that most processed food comes with a standardized nutrition label. You're lucky, you're beginning to read labels just when it has become a lot easier. In the 1990s the government standardized all food labels and checks to make sure such claims as low salt are really what they mean.

Serving Size

Is your serving the same size as the one on the label? Remember if you double the serving size, you're eating double the grams of fat, sodium, carbohydrates, and proteins. Serving size is *very* important. Imagine that you're reading the nutrition label for a box of Ritz crackers. If it lists a serving as *three* crackers, and *each one* contains 3 grams of fat, a sleeve of them (which is what people usually eat) would equal all the fat you'd want to eat in one day. Most companies don't make up ridiculous serving sizes, but keep your eyes open. What doesn't seem like a lot to you may be five to ten servings.

Nutrition Facts

Serving Size ½ cup (114g)

Servings Per Container 4

Amount Per Serving

Calories 90	Calories from Fat 30

	% Daily Value*
Total Fat 3g	**5%**
Saturated Fat 0g	**0%**
Cholesterol 0mg	**0%**
Sodium 300mg	**13%**
Total Carbohydrate 13g	**4%**
Dietary Fiber 3g	**12%**
Sugars 3g	
Protein 3g	

Vitamin A	80%	•	Vitamin C	60%
Calcium	4%	•	Iron	4%

* Percent Daily Values are based on a 2,000
calorie diet. Your daily values may be higher or
lower depending on your calorie needs:

	Calories	2,000	2,600
Total Fat	Less than	65g	80g
Sat. Fat	Less than	20g	25g
Cholesterol	Less than	300mg	300mg
Sodium	Less than	2,400mg	2,400mg
Total Carbohydrate		300g	375g
Fiber		25g	30g

Calories per gram:

Fat 9	•	Carbohydrate 4	•	Protein 4

More nutrients may be listed on some labels.

Calories

The total calories, for each serving of the food, includes all the fat, sugar, protein, and carbohydrate calories. Just because something is fat free does *not* mean it is low in calories. A 5-foot 4-inch, 138-pound active woman needs 2,200 calories a day. A 5-foot 10-inch, 174-pound man needs 2,900. If you're trying to lose weight you need even less. Watch your fat, but don't become blind to calories either.

Dietary Fiber

Fiber is especially important in keeping your body running at top speed. And it fills you up, keeping you from eating more fats and sugars.

Total Fat

Aim low: Most people need to cut back on fat. Women should eat approximately 40 to 50 grams of fat a day; men should eat approximately 50 to 65. For a healthy diet and a healthy body, choose foods with a big difference between the total number of calories and the number of calories from fat.

Daily Value

Do you feel that there are far too many numbers to keep track of? Let the daily value be your guide. The values are listed for people who eat 2,000 or 2,500 calories a day. For fat, saturated fat, cholesterol, sugar, and sodium, you want to choose foods that have very low daily values. For dietary fiber, potassium, and other vitamins and minerals you want to reach 100 percent every day, and here you don't have to worry about going over!

Lurking Sodium in Your Food

Sodium Sources	In Foods
1. salt (sodium chloride)	cooking, at the table, processing
2. monosodium glutamate (MSG)	seasoning, in Asian food, TV dinners
3. baking powder	quick breads, cakes, pastries, cookies
4. baking soda (sodium bicarbonate)	breads and cakes, alkalizer for indigestion
5. brine	corned beef, pickles, sauerkraut
6. sodium propionate	pasteurized cheeses; as a preservative in some breads and cakes to inhibit mold growth
7. disodium phosphate	quick-cooking cereal and processed cheeses
8. sodium alginate	chocolate milk, ice cream
9. sodium benzoate	relishes, sauces, dressings
10. sodium hydroxide	ripe olives, pretzels, hominy, some processed fruits and vegetables
11. sodium nitrate and sodium nitrite	cured meats
12. sodium sulfite	maraschino cherries, glazed or crystallized fruit, dried fruit
13. sodium caseinate	ice cream, frozen custard
14. sodium citrate	gelatin desserts, beverages
15. sodium pectinate	syrups for ice cream, sherbet, fruit jelly, salad dressing
16. sodium saccharin	soft drinks, artificial sweeteners

Sodium

Be particularly cautious about sodium. An average person can eat 1,100 to 3,300 grams of sodium a day. Stick to foods lower in sodium and salt. The nutrition label will give you definite numbers, but the rest of the packaging may be plastered with other claims. If the box says sodium free or no sodium—it contains less than 5 milligrams per serving. If it says it is very low sodium—it contains 35 milligrams or less per serving. If it's low sodium —it has 140 milligrams or less per serving.

If a food says that it's lower in sodium than its regular version, it can still be high in sodium. Reduced sodium means it is processed to reduce the usual level of sodium by 75 percent, and note that the label *must* identify the comparison food. If it says unsalted, or no salt added, or without added salt—it's been processed without salt—*but* it may still contain sodium that is naturally present in your food.

Sodium lurks in your food through many different processing techniques. Follow your nutrition labels, and take some time to read the ingredients of some of your foods. You'd be surprised at all the extra sodium. The list on page 57 shows some of the ways sodium finds its way into your body, all without your even touching a saltshaker.

In the Kitchen

First, learn to cook. Even knowing a few simple dishes can help you keep your sodium down. There are literally hundreds of cookbooks in the bookstore and right there in the grocery store racks are healthy food magazines. From Betty Crocker to *Vegetarian Times*, they are full of low-sodium, low-fat dishes you can make fast. Especially keep your eye out for vegetable recipes that make your mouth water. It's just another way to get your three to five servings a day.

When you are cooking, start by cutting the

amount of salt you add in half, working your way toward not adding any salt at all. It will usually make very little difference in the taste of your foods, especially once your taste buds have adapted to your lower salt diet. Spice salt substitutes, like Mrs. Dash, add extra flavor to your food and give you that satisfaction of "shaking" onto your food, but without the dangers of salt. Also try substituting vinegar in recipes that need a "kick" and add a splash shaker to your table. Vinegar gives the extra tang flavor that salt does.

In Chapter 8 you'll find some innovative ways to adapt your favorite recipes and some tasty recipes to get you started cooking healthily.

Chapter Six

Eating Out

There are usually two main reasons not to eat at home. One, you're in a hurry and you're hungry. Two, you're going to a sit-down restaurant for an occasion. Eating healthy is quite different at both places. At a fast-food stop, your primary interest is getting good tasting food quickly and continuing on. If you eat out often, it's important to choose low-fat foods; if you eat out only on special occasions, then splurging is definitely acceptable. At a sit-down restaurant, your interests may vary from conducting a business meal to celebrating an occasion. You might initially feel self-conscious, but you'll discover it may in fact be easier to make healthy choices in a restaurant, because there's a wide selection of foods and you can specify such special things as low salt.

As you see, there are always two ways to look at what you're eating.

Fast Food

The key to eating healthy fast food is to make quick easy choices. Almost all fast food chains provide nutritional information, and if you eat at them often, it's worth your time to ask the manager for it. The result may surprise you. For example, here's two sample lunches at McDonald's.

	Calories	Fat (grams)	Sodium (mg)
Quarter Pounder			
with Cheese	517	29	1,150
Small Fries	220	12	110
Apple Pie	262	15	240
Total	999	56	1,500
OR			
Hamburger	257	10	460
Chunky Chicken			
Salad	141	3	230
Lite Vinaigrette	15	1	60
Low-fat Vanilla			
Shake	290	1	170
Total	703	15	920

Surprise—the apple pie has more sodium than the French fries! Of course, the amount doesn't account for the salt added to the French fries. The total fat in the first meal is around the recommended amount of fat you should eat *all day*. But the second meal shows how you *can* make healthy choices in fast food if you choose wisely. What's even more surprising than the fat or sodium is that you get *much more* food in the second, healthier choice.

What fast food often lacks is vegetables. Your choices are usually fried potatoes, buttery mashed potatoes, or baked potatoes with butter, sour cream, bacon, *and* chili. Salads are often a healthy alternative, but adding cheese and heavy dressings makes them less of a positive choice.

Chicken and fish sandwiches are often a pleasant alternative to burgers. But as soon as they hit the deep fryer, they're often higher in fat and sodium than your hamburger. The breading and seasoning often used on fried foods are also usually very high in salt. Grilled and rotisserie chicken is much lower in fat, but is usually marinated so make sure to ask if the marinade is high in salt. Broiled fish, available at most Long John Silver's and other fast food places, is also a better choice. But stay away from the high-fat and high-salt tartar sauce and cocktail sauce. A brisk shake of pepper and lemon juice is usually all the seasoning you need.

French fries can never really be low-fat at a fast food restaurant, but if you really can't go without them, save them for every other trip, and get small servings without added salt or ketchup. If they're so good you can't go without them, enjoy their taste slowly and eat them one by one, or share the serving with someone else.

Hot dogs have an exceptionally high amount of fat and sodium. Even turkey or chicken dogs are high in fat. Save hot dogs for special occasions when they're really perfect—a baseball game, an outdoor grill. Or choose the new lower-fat hot dog; you probably won't even be able to taste the difference.

Tacos are usually very high in fat and salt, with fatty, salty seasoned beef, cheese, sour cream, and a salted, fried tortilla shell. But now there are some good choices at fast-food Mexican restaurants. In general, flour tortillas are better choices than fried corn tortillas. Most flour tortillas in fast-food restaurants are made without lard, but if you're not sure, just ask. Avoid high-fat cheese and sour cream, but pile on the lettuce, tomatoes, and whole beans. Refried beans can be a good choice, but ask if they're made with extra lard or oil. Salsa, like ketchup, is very high in salt, and so are jalapeños, so again, save them until you really want them and use smaller amounts. Some Mexican restaurants have "light" selections that use low-fat sour cream and cheeses. These are wonderful choices; just make sure to look over the *actual* fat and sodium counts to verify that *their* version of low salt and low fat is the same as yours.

Fast Chinese and Japanese food can be wonderful for your diet or a disaster. Stay away from fried rice, eggrolls, tempura, and dishes described as crispy. Remember Japan and China have the highest levels of sodium and the highest levels of high blood pressure. Soy sauce and MSG are often the high-salt culprits. If you adore Asian food on your lunch hour, keep a shaker of low-sodium soy sauce at your desk or in your locker. Chinese restaurants are now used to people requesting no MSG; take the extra step and ask if they have low-sodium soy sauce also. Wonderful for your diet is steamed rice, bonus points if it's brown rice, sushi, steamed fresh vegetables, tofu, or stir-fried vegetables in small amounts of oil. Since sauce is usually loaded with fat and sodium, one suggestion is to lift foods out using chopsticks or forks so you use less sauce.

Thai food and noodle houses are becoming more common. The same rules apply; ask if the seasoning is salty, if the dish is fried. Thai food involves less soy sauce, but similar salty sauces replace it, such as nam pla, and Thai cooking usually involves more saturated fat as cooking oil and in coconut milk. But on the whole, Thai food is very light and flavorful.

Indian and Middle Eastern foods are quite often very good choices for low-salt and low-fat foods. The interesting spices used are unusual to most Americans, and give richer flavors than salt. Make sure you ask about the ingredients, and on your own, taste food for its saltiness.

Deli meats such as pastrami, corned beef, bologna, are often high in fat and salt. Choose non-cured or smoked meats such as turkey and roast beef. Ask for a smaller portion of meat, stick to three ounces, hold the mayo and cheese and pile on all the veggies you like. Unfortunately, many of the prepared salads at delis are very high in salt and fat. One quick question, "Do you have any 'lighter' salads?" isn't being too picky and just about every place that sells food now has lighter, healthier options. And remember you can work in high-salt items such as deli pickles. But choose wisely; skip salty snacks such as popcorn and pretzels and you're free to eat a pickle at lunch. You're not keeping yourself from eating foods you love, you're *juggling* them.

Dining Out

It's impossible to list all the reasons people eat in restaurants. To experience different foods, business meetings, anniversaries, weddings, and to enjoy someone's company are just a few reasons. Food permeates all social functions. The key to eating healthily is the same as in fast food—*choose wisely*.

When your menu arrives see it as an opportunity to experiment, to taste new ways of preparing vegetables or fish, two of the most challenging things to cook at home. If you wish, dive into the complimentary basket of bread, leaving the butter behind or using very, very little. Remember that with every meal you're trying to follow the daily food pyramid—heavy on the complex carbohydrates, fruits and vegetables, lower on meat and dairy, and very light on fats and sugars.

Begin your meal with a fruit plate or a small salad with the dressing on the side. Be brave! Ordering dressing on the side is so common no one even thinks twice about it. Unfortunately, most soups are very salty and heavy on the cream, so it's usually best to stick to a fruit or vegetable appetizer.

For your main dish, look for meats that are seared, grilled, broiled, or poached. As always, foods that are fried, or pickled will be high in fat and sodium.

The most luxurious part of dining out is being able to tailor your meal to what you *want* to eat. Special requests are almost the norm in most restaurants, and you're paying for this meal, so don't be shy. Even the snooty waiter would rather you told him beforehand that you wanted extra vegetables and no salt than if you sent the food back. Speak up and ask questions about the food. How is it prepared? Is there cream or extra salt in this dish?

It's perfectly acceptable to order a light rice or

vegetable side dish as an appetizer. In fact, restaurants are now quite used to their patrons ordering appetizers as their dinners. One of the most notable things about dining out is the mammoth portions. If you're comfortable with the idea, plan on taking half your dinner home. It's quite an acceptable practice, and because you're there to enjoy the food anyway, you'll want to eat it again later.

The amount of questions or changes you ask depends solely on how comfortable you feel. If you're a guest at a large business dinner, you probably won't want to make the waiter answer hundreds of questions. But if you're out with your family you'll be more free to ask for more changes and special items.

In certain situations, such as weddings, airplane trips, or some business events, your food has already been ordered for you. Sometimes you will have the opportunity to call ahead and make special arrangements. The best and easiest way to order a special meal is to simply ask for a vegetarian plate. If you call ahead, there's no uncomfortable wait to change your order while everyone else is eating, and most likely, *your* food will be better than everyone else's.

There are lots of times when you simply can't or don't want to make special arrangements for your meal. Never feel guilty for a "night off." If you make your diet stringent and rigid, you'll most likely rebel, stuff yourself with unhealthy foods and never try to eat healthily again and feel guilty about your lack of willpower. You're beginning a way of life— but don't forget to live! Eating one meal will *not* put you in the hospital. One bag of potato chips doesn't mean you are a *bad* person; it simply means you ate a bag of potato chips. Tomorrow don't eat a bag of potato chips. Tomorrow eat a lighter lunch and dinner. And congratulate yourself afterward. You're striving toward a diet *balance*. By letting yourself eat what you want sometimes, you'll be more likely to be healthy overall.

Chapter Seven

Weight Control

Surveys have found that up to 60 percent of hypertensive people are obese. This isn't surprising when, on average, overweight adults have a three times greater risk of "catching" hypertension than people with normal weight. One possible reason why obese people have higher blood pressures is that the extra weight requires that the heart work harder to supply blood to the excess tissue.

If you're overweight, the best thing you can do to lower your blood pressure is to lose weight. Often blood pressure drops dramatically when overweight people lose weight. Even losing two to five pounds can help you lower your blood pressure enough to allow you to stop taking pills.

Successful weight control is a lifelong commitment. You need to set realistic goals for slow, steady weight loss, no more than one to two pounds a week. By eating less fat and fewer calories and by adopting behavior modification strategies to deal with high-risk emotional and social situations, you're making changes for the rest of your life.

The first question participants going through the nutrition programs at Stedman Center ask is "How much weight can I lose and how fast can I do it?" Fads such as very-low-calorie diets, liquid diets, and diet pills are not the answer. Most people regain all they've lost and often even gain *more* weight shortly after going off such diets. These regimens are impractical for long-term weight control, probably expensive, may be dangerous to your health, and may lead to negative eating behaviors.

The National Institutes of Health convened an expert panel to discuss the safety and effectiveness of weight-loss techniques. They concluded that:

1. Liquid diets and other "very-low-calorie" programs (fewer than 1,200 calories a day) are dangerous; such programs should be reserved for the very obese and be supervised by a physician.
2. Chronic dieting is actually an eating disorder, like anorexia or bulimia. Americans, especially women, are being held to an impossibly ideal body image. We would be better off physically and emotionally if we learned to eat in a more natural, spontaneous, and balanced way.

The most effective way to lose weight forever is to have a balanced low-fat diet and adopt some form of moderate exercise.

By using strategies we recommend in this book, many people have successfully lost weight and kept it off for years. We believe you can too.

Suggested Weight for Adults		
Height	Weight	
	19–34 years	*> 35 years*
5′	97–128	108–138
5′1″	101–132	111–143
5′2″	104–137	115–148
5′3″	107–141	119–152
5′4″	111–146	122–157
5′5″	114–150	126–162
5′6″	118–155	130–167
5′7″	121–160	134–172
5′8″	125–164	138–178
5′9″	129–169	142–183
5′10″	132–174	146–188
5′11″	136–179	151–194
6′	140–184	155–199
6′1″	144–189	159–205
6′2″	148–195	164–210
6′3″	152–200	168–216
6′4″	156–205	173–222
6′5″	160–211	177–228
6′6″	164–216	182–234

Data from the Dietary Guidelines for Americans, U.S. Department of Health and Human Services, 1990.

Your Health Assessment

First things first—you need to know where you stand. Everyone is different and so is everyone's hypertension. To make *your* high blood pressure go down we need to develop a program perfect for *you.*

In general, your weight should be toward the lower end of the ranges if you are a woman. The higher rates apply to men because overall they have more muscle and bone than women. Although this table should apply to most people, *definitely* consult your physician or other health professional for the *achievable* and *maintainable* weight for *you.*

Waist-to-Hip Ratio

While being overweight is a health risk, the *way* you carry your extra weight also has implications for your health. The waist-to-hip ratio appears to have a better correlation with heart disease than other weight measurements. Scientists believe that people who have their extra weight around their abdomen, "apples," are at greater risk for heart disease than "pears," who store their extra fat around their hips.

A waist-to-hip ratio greater than 1.0 for men and 0.8 for women indicates increased cardiac risk, states the American Heart Association.

If your waist-to-hip ratio is high you are an "apple" and have even more reason to lose weight. Carrying your extra weight around your stomach means there's more fat around your vital organs. The strain on these organs—your heart, liver, kidneys—increases the number of health problems you'll have. By following your new healthy way to live, you should see a difference in your weight, your blood pressure, and how you feel.

If your waist-to-hip ratio is low, then you are a "pear," which means you store more fat in the buttocks, thighs, and hips. Although this pattern of fat distribution does not add more risk (than you already have from being overweight), these fat tissues are less active metabolically and may be more difficult to take off. (Except for lactating women, who are able to lose added weight around their hips and thighs quickly.)

Finding Your Waist-to-Hip Ratio

Step #1: Using a tape measure, find the circumference of your waist at its narrowest point when your stomach is relaxed.

waist = _____ in.

Step #2: Next, measure the circumference of your hips at their widest (where your buttocks protrude the most)

hips = _____ in.

Step #3: Finally, divide your waist measurement by your hips measurement

$$\frac{waist}{hips} = \text{waist-to-hip ratio}$$

The waist-to-hip ratio may also partially explain the difference in high blood pressure between men and women. Men are more likely to be "apples" and women to be "pears." This may be part of the reason why men have higher rates of hypertension and more complications. So how do you go about losing some weight? Slowly.

Body weight remains constant when the amount of calories you eat equals the amount of calories you expend through living. Therefore, to lose weight, you can either eat fewer calories or increase the amount of calories you expend or a combination of both. Roughly, to lose one pound of weight, you need to create a calorie deficit of 3,500 kilocalories. We recommend that you either reduce the amount of calories you eat or increase your expenditure of calories by about 500 kilocalories a day. Although this may not give you fast weight loss, this will lead to about one pound of weight loss a week. Remember, the exact rate may vary according to the individual. As explained earlier, if you decrease fat intake, increase whole grains, fruit, and vegetables, you are likely to eat fewer calories as well. Small changes can make a big difference and last a long time.

An accurate food diary can help identify problems in your eating habits. By writing down what you eat in one typical day, you give yourself an idea of *what* you eat, *where*, and *why*. You can also find out extra sources of calories, fat, or sodium that are often overlooked. One of the easiest ways to keep a food diary is to carry a few blank index cards in your pocket. After you eat, write down what you've eaten and include all the small ingredients, such as ketchup, dressing, beverages, and snacks. Don't try to impress yourself by changing the usual way you eat because you want to assess your true eating behavior. In your food diary, don't forget to include unconscious eating, "when the calories don't count." Some examples are: eating while cooking, eating while cleaning up, nibbling off other people's plates, and "leveling" the cake. Begin to focus on awareness when eating—what does the food look like, smell like, taste like? Are you physically hungry? Compare your diary to what we recommend in Chapter 4 and evaluate yourself to see how you are doing and what you can do to improve.

Once you start making changes in your diet, keeping a food diary periodically will also help you monitor your progress, see where you stand, and tell you where you can make more changes. Along with the food diary, you can also keep track of your progress in other areas, such as changes in your blood pressure, cholesterol, weight, and how your clothes fit.

The key to having a healthy diet (which in turn promotes weight loss) involves combining the science of nutrition (low-fat/sodium, increase in fruits and vegetables) and the art of eating (eating for hunger, not using food as a crutch). Food is not just fuel for our bodies but fuel for our celebrations, fuel for our boredom, fuel for our anxieties, fuel for our stress. The process of changing our eating behavior is long and requires time and effort. Following Stedman's strategies, you can start the process of following and enjoying a balanced diet.

Part of this process to normalize eating is to become more aware of the physical signs of hunger (hunger pangs/pain, dizziness, headache, nausea) and the physical signs of being full or stuffed (bloating, a tight feeling, loosening your belt, nausea). The goal is to teach yourself how to feel *satisfied* instead of stuffed or starved. The purpose of understanding hunger is to realize the difference between physical hunger and emotional hunger. Attempt to understand why you eat when you're not *physically* hungry and you can start down the road to balanced, healthy eating.

If you begin to notice that emotional eating is a problem for you, get some additional help. Changing any behavior, from quitting cigarettes to teaching yourself not to eat when you're lonely, is *very* difficult. Get help from support groups, psychologists, dietitians, and social workers. *Never* feel that food is controlling you. You can eat what you want when you want it. Have patience; it will take a few years for you to learn *healthy* ways to eat.

Exercise

The American Heart Association recently recognized inactivity as the fourth major risk factor for heart disease, along with being overweight, hypertension, and cigarette smoking. As you can see, if you have hypertension, are overweight, don't exercise, and smoke, you're setting yourself up for a big painful fall.

Most American adults get little or no physical activity. Lack of regular exercise causes 12 percent of all deaths in the United States, 250,000 deaths a year. Exercise will help you lose weight by changing your basal metabolism and making you feel better about yourself. Research has shown that people who exercise and follow a healthy diet are much more likely to lose weight and keep it off.

Think about how much exercise you did yesterday. Did you include walking your dog, cleaning the bathroom, taking two to three flights of stairs? In February 1995 the American College of Sports Medicine and the Centers for Disease Control and Prevention came out with a new joint recommendation for physical activity: that every adult get 30 minutes or more of moderate-intensity physical activity on most, and preferably all, days of the week. The 30 minutes can be accumulated intermittently and can include such activities as raking leaves and cleaning the house.

You *don't* have to rush out and buy expensive health club memberships or equipment. The key to incorporating exercise into your life forever is just that—incorporation. Consult with your physician before starting an exercise program. Figure out a modest commitment that you can stick to, get a partner, be in a class, try activities such as bicycling and dancing. Not every exercise is a strict, regimented regime where you "work out" for 30 minutes and then drive one block to the convenience store to buy milk. Do whatever works for *you*. If you like taking classes, do so. If you like walking around your neighborhood, do so. Exercising will make you *feel* healthier and encourage your healthy eating. Make sure you drink lots of water and keep fruit and vegetable snacks around after you exercise, a positive reinforcement for your healthy lifestyle.

And as an added benefit, let your insurance company and human resources department in your office know that you're taking better care of your health. Many companies will pay for your exercise classes and insurance companies may lower your yearly premiums.

Chapter Eight

Recipes

Modify Your Favorites and
Experience New Tastes

For lower fat and cholesterol in your favorite recipes use the following substitutions:

> Whole milk—use skim or nonfat milk.
>
> Cream—use evaporated skim milk
>
> Creamed soups—use ½ can of creamy soup and ½ can of skim milk
>
> Sour cream—if you're putting sour cream in a hot dish, use nonfat plain yogurt with one tablespoon of flour mixed in for each cup to prevent the yogurt from separating;
>
> —if you're using cold sour cream on food, like topping a baked potato, use the Mock Sour Cream recipe on page 115;
>
> —use pureed low-fat cottage cheese.

Main Dishes

Spinach-Stuffed Shells

This dish feeds 10! It is perfect for freezing and thaw-ing for quick dinners later and can even be warmed in a toaster oven.

Spinach Filling

1	cup diced onions
1	cup chopped scallions
1	teaspoon olive oil
3	pounds chopped frozen spinach, defrosted
¼	cup chopped parsley
¼	cup chopped fresh dill (optional)
¼	cup grated parmesan
1½	cups grated mozzarella (part skim)
¾	cup low-fat cottage cheese
3	egg whites
½	teaspoon black pepper

Sauté the onions and scallions in the olive oil until the onions are sweet and translucent. Squeeze the defrosted spinach like a sponge to remove excess water. In a large bowl mix the spinach and the sautéed onions and scallions with all the other ingredients.

Yield: 15 ⅓-cup servings

Calories per serving: 78
Fat: 2.6 g.
Sodium: 208 mg.

You can use this spinach mixture for many other recipes, including putting it into a pie crust for spinach pie, using different noodles and making lasagna, making a stuffing for bell peppers, and stuffing fish.

For Shells

1	pound pasta shells
2	cups tomato sauce
5	cups Spinach Filling

Cook the pasta shells until they are al dente. In a casserole dish spread out 1½ cups of the tomato sauce. Fill each shell with 2 tablespoons of the spinach filling and place in the casserole dish. Pour the remaining tomato sauce over the shells and cover loosely with aluminum foil. Cook for 20 minutes in a preheated 350°F. oven.

Yield: 10 servings

Calories per serving: 301
Fat: 5.4 g.
Sodium: 343 mg.

Moroccan Vegetable Stew

Here is another recipe that is perfect for freezing and eating later. It also makes a great hearty lunch if you can use a microwave at work.

1	cup kidney beans
2	bay leaves
1½	teaspoons olive oil
2	cups red bell peppers, diced into large chunks
3	cups onions, diced into large chunks
4	cloves garlic, minced
¾	teaspoon ground cumin
1¾	teaspoons ground coriander seeds
1½	teaspoons curry powder
1½	teaspoons salt
6½	cups zucchini, diced into large chunks
1	2-pound can low-sodium Italian-style tomatoes
4	cups squash (butternut, acorn, pumpkin), peeled and diced into large chunks
1½	pounds potatoes, diced into large chunks

In a small saucepan heat the kidney beans with the bay leaves; take out the bay leaves and set aside. Heat the olive oil in a large pot and lightly sauté the peppers, onions, and garlic. Once they are hot, add everything else—the kidney beans, seasonings, zucchini, tomatoes (use the liquid, too), squash, and potatoes. As soon as the potatoes are soft, the stew is ready to eat.

Yield: 12 ¾-cup servings

Calories per serving: 181
Fat: 1.3 g.
Sodium: 287 mg.

Chicken Stir-Fry

½   cup sliced onions
½   cup sliced green peppers
½   cup yellow squash (half rounds)
½   teaspoon sesame oil
4   ounces cooked chicken
1   teaspoon rice vinegar
1   teaspoon low-salt soy sauce
½   cup broccoli florets
1   cup cooked brown rice
2   tablespoons water or stock

In a nonstick sauté pan, sauté the onions, peppers, and squash in the sesame oil. When the vegetables are soft, add the chicken and cook until heated through. Add the rice vinegar, soy sauce, and broccoli. Cover and let steam until the broccoli is lightly cooked, 2 to 3 minutes. Meanwhile, heat the rice in a separate pan, adding water to prevent scorching. Serve the chicken mixture over the rice.

Yield: 2 servings

Calories per serving: 248
Fat: 4.3 g.
Sodium: 313 mg.

Chicken with Saffron Rice

¾	pound skinless, boneless chicken breast
2	tablespoons flour
⅛	teaspoon cumin
⅛	teaspoon coriander seeds
⅛	teaspoon salt
⅛	teaspoon pepper
2	teaspoons olive oil
1	cup chopped onions
1	clove garlic, minced
⅛	teaspoon saffron
2	cups chicken stock
	dash of Tabasco
1	cup white rice
1	cup chopped tomatoes
1½	cups frozen peas
¼	cup chopped parsley

Cut the chicken into 1-inch-wide strips. Combine the flour, cumin, coriander, salt, and pepper. Dredge the chicken in the flour-spice mixture and sauté in the olive oil. Take out the chicken and set it on paper towels to drain. In the same pan sauté the onions and garlic. Add the saffron and 1 cup of chicken stock. Deglaze the pan. Transfer the onions, garlic, saffron, and chicken stock into a saucepan; add the remaining 1 cup chicken stock and the Tabasco; add the rice and cover tightly. Cook for about 10 minutes, or until the rice is done. In a large bowl mix together the chicken, the rice mixture, the tomatoes, peas, and half the parsley, and place in a casserole dish. Cover and heat through. Sprinkle with the remaining parsley before serving.

Yield: 10 ¾-cup servings

Calories per serving: 182
Fat: 1.8 g.
Sodium: 121 mg.

Grilled Chicken

1	clove garlic
1½	tablespoons Dijon mustard
1	tablespoon fresh rosemary
1¼	pounds chicken breast

Crush the garlic and mix with the next two ingredients. Marinate the chicken in the mixture, turning occasionally, overnight in the refrigerator. Grill outdoors or under broiler for 5 minutes, or until done.

Yield: 6 3-ounce servings

Calories per serving: 98
Fat: 1.2 g.
Sodium: 104 mg.

Roast Turkey Breast

¼   cup peanut oil
3   tablespoons lemon juice
½   cup white wine
4   cloves garlic, minced
2   teaspoons thyme
1   teaspoon hot pepper flakes
1   boneless turkey breast, with skin,
    approximately 3 pounds

Combine the oil, lemon juice, white wine, garlic, thyme, and hot pepper flakes and pour over the turkey breast. Let marinate for 4 hours in the refrigerator. Remove the breast from the marinade, place on a baking sheet, and brown under the broiler flesh side up, then turn and brown skin side up. Remove from the broiler, pour the marinade over the breast, and finish cooking in a 350°F. oven for about 30 minutes.

Yield: 12 3-ounce servings

Calories per serving: 214
Fat: 6 g.
Sodium: 78 mg.

Pearl Balls

½ cup Chinese "sticky" rice
⅔ pound ground turkey
½ teaspoon salt
½ teaspoon sherry
½ teaspoon black pepper
2 tablespoons water
1 tablespoon cornstarch

Cover the rice with water and soak for 2 hours. Mix the remaining ingredients and form into 1-inch balls. Spread the rice onto a clean plate. Roll the meatballs over the rice until covered. Steam the balls for 20 minutes. Serve warm.

Yield: 15 servings (serving size: 2 balls)

Calories per serving: 80
Fat: 1.98 g.
Sodium: 88.8 mg.

Baked Catfish

⅓ cup white flour
⅓ cup bread crumbs
1½ teaspoons paprika
    dash of black pepper
2 tablespoons grated parmesan
2 8-ounce fillets catfish
¾ cup plain yogurt
    cooking spray

Preheat the oven to 450°F. Mix the flour, bread crumbs, paprika, pepper, and parmesan. Cut the fish into 5-ounce pieces. Coat with the yogurt and dredge in the flour/bread crumb mixture. Place on sheet pans lightly sprayed with nonstick spray. Bake for 10 minutes.

Yield: 4 3-ounce servings

Calories per serving: 274
Fat: 8 g.
Sodium: 244 mg.

Sesame Mahimahi

1   teaspoon sesame oil
1   tablespoon rice wine vinegar
2   teaspoons soy sauce
2   5-ounce mahimahi fillets
1   teaspoon sesame seeds

Combine the oil, vinegar, and soy sauce and pour over the fish. Bake in a shallow pan in a preheated 400°F. oven for 8 to 10 minutes. To toast the sesame seeds: place the sesame seeds on a cookie sheet and bake for 4 to 5 minutes in a 375°F. oven, until brown. Sprinkle on top of the fish.

Yield: 2 servings

Calories per serving: 188
Fat: 6.3 g.
Sodium: 220 mg.

Salmon Cakes

2	tablespoons nonfat plain yogurt
1¼	pounds salmon fillets
1	egg white
½	cup onion, minced
¼	cup chopped green pepper
¼	cup chopped scallions
2	teaspoons mustard
¼	cup flour
1	tablespoon peanut oil

Set the yogurt in a coffee filter and allow to drain for at least 2 hours. (One-half cup yogurt will yield at least 2 tablespoons.) Chop ¼ pound salmon into ½-inch pieces and set aside. Process the remaining 1 pound salmon in a food processor, add to the reserved salmon pieces, and mix in the egg white. Stir in the onion, pepper, scallions, and mustard. Carefully fold in the yogurt. Scoop out six ½-cup servings onto a baking sheet that has been lightly dusted with one-half the flour. Sprinkle the tops of the patties with the remaining flour. Heat a nonstick sauté pan, add 1 teaspoon oil, and gently brown each side of two patties. Set on a clean baking sheet and lightly sauté the remaining salmon cakes in the rest of the oil. When done, bake the salmon cakes in a preheated 350°F. oven for approximately 10 minutes.

Yield: 6 cakes

Calories per cake: 187
Fat: 9 g.
Sodium: 81 mg.

Baked Grouper

¼   cup rice vinegar
2   tablespoons light soy sauce
2   teaspoons sesame oil
2   teaspoons minced gingerroot
1   clove garlic, minced
6   5-ounce grouper fillets
    cooking spray
1   lime, sliced
¼   cup chopped scallions

Combine the vinegar, soy sauce, sesame oil, ginger, and garlic, pour over the grouper, and refrigerator for 1 hour. Preheat the oven to 450°F. Place the marinated fish pieces on a baking sheet lightly sprayed with cooking spray. Pour the marinade over the fish and bake for 7 to 10 minutes. Serve with slices of lime and scallions sprinkled on top.

Yield: 6 3-ounce servings

Calories per serving: 159
Fat: 3.3 g.
Sodium: 200 mg.

Flounder Stuffed with Mushrooms

8   ounces mushrooms, sliced
⅓   cup sliced scallions
½   teaspoon minced fresh ginger
1   teaspoon olive oil
4   dried shiitake mushrooms
2   tablespoons chopped parsley
1   tablespoon lemon juice
     black pepper
4   5-ounce flounder fillets
⅓   cup water or white wine

Sauté the mushrooms, scallions, and ginger in the olive oil. To rehydrate the shiitake mushrooms: Cover with boiling water, let sit for 5 minutes, then drain; slice and add to the sautéed mixture. Remove from the heat and add the parsley. Sprinkle the lemon and black pepper on the fish fillets. To stuff: Place 1 tablespoon stuffing at end of each fillet and roll up. Place the fish in a shallow baking dish and add the water or wine. Bake in a preheated 350°F. oven for 25 minutes, or until the fish is done.

Yield: 4 servings

Calories per serving: 161
Fat: 3.1 g.
Sodium: 119 mg.

Shrimp Scampi

¾	cup sliced carrots
¾	cup snow peas
2	cloves garlic, minced
2	cups chicken stock
2	tablespoons lemon juice
2	tablespoons cornstarch
3	tablespoons buttermilk
1½	tablespoons grated parmesan
	dash of white pepper
2	tablespoons chopped parsley
½	pound linguini
1	pound shrimp, shelled
1	lemon, cut into 6 wedges

Steam the carrots for 2 minutes and set aside. Steam the snow peas for 30 seconds and hold. Meanwhile, make the sauce by combining the garlic, chicken stock, and lemon juice. Bring to a boil, add the cornstarch, which has been dissolved in the buttermilk. Add the parmesan, pepper, and 1 tablespoon chopped parsley, and simmer until the sauce has a liquid consistency. Cook the linguini until al dente, drain, and add to the sauce. Steam the shrimp for 3 minutes. Add the vegetables to the sauce and place the pasta, sauce, and vegetables, on a serving plate.

Top with the shrimp and garnish with the remaining chopped parsley and lemon wedges.

Yield: 6 ¾-cup servings

Calories per serving: 166
Fat: 2 g.
Sodium: 259 mg.

Shrimp and Green Peas

4	teaspoons cornstarch
10	large shrimp, shelled and cleaned
2	teaspoons dry white wine
⅛	teaspoon salt
1	teaspoon canola oil
3	cloves garlic
1	teaspoon ground ginger
¾	cup green peas

Mix the cornstarch, wine, and salt into a smooth paste; then toss the shrimp in until covered completely. Heat the oil in a skillet. Lightly stir-fry the garlic and ginger. Toss the peas and shrimp in the pan. Stir-fry until the peas are tender and the shrimp turns translucent. Serve with steamed rice and vegetables on a large serving dish.

Yield: 2 servings

Calories per serving: 111
Fat: 2.7 g.
Sodium: 227 mg.

Beef Chili

¼	pound dry red kidney beans
1¼	pounds beef round, cut into 1-inch cubes
½	tablespoon olive oil
¾	cup diced onions
1	clove garlic, minced
¾	cup diced green peppers
1½	cups canned tomatoes
1	teaspoon dried basil
½	tablespoon chili powder
½	tablespoon ground cumin

Rinse the beans, place in a 2-quart pot, and cover with water. Boil, remove from the heat, cover tightly with a lid, and let sit for 1 hour. Put back on the stove, bring to a boil, then simmer until the beans are soft. Drain and reserve. Sauté the beef in the olive oil in a heavy bottomed pot until brown. Add the onions and garlic and cook until the onions are translucent. Add the peppers and tomatoes with the liquid. Bring to a boil, then simmer until the beef is tender, about 40 minutes. Add the remaining spices and the cooked beans.

Yield: 16 ½-cup servings

Calories per serving: 212
Fat: 6.9 g.
Sodium: 188 mg.

Marinated Flank Steak

½ cup reduced-calorie Italian dressing
2 tablespoons lemon juice
2 tablespoons vinegar (try herb,
   balsamic, or wine vinegar)
¼ teaspoon garlic powder
1 pound flank steak or other lean steak

Combine all the ingredients except the steak and mix well. Marinate the steak in the mixture in a flat-covered dish for at least 24 hours and up to 72 hours in the refrigerator. Turn the steak occasionally. Broil or grill on high to a rare degree of doneness (about 3 to 4 minutes per side). Slice thin across the grain of the meat.

Yield: 4 servings

Calories per serving: 180
Fat: 5 g.
Sodium: 300 mg.

Honey-Mustard Tenderloin

1   whole pork tenderloin, about 1 pound
4   tablespoons honey
2   tablespoons cider vinegar
2   tablespoons brown sugar
1   tablespoon Dijon mustard
½   teaspoon paprika

Preheat the oven to 375°F. Trim all visible fat from the meat. Combine the remaining ingredients thoroughly. Coat the tenderloin well with the sauce. Roast at 375°F. for 20 to 30 minutes, basting occasionally, until a meat thermometer registers 160°F. Slice thin to serve.

Yield: 4 servings

Calories per serving: 229
Fat: 4 g.
Sodium: 80 mg.

Vegetable
Dishes

Stuffed Peppers

You can use red, green, or yellow peppers; the red and yellow are sweeter tasting and more expensive. You can also stuff the peppers with the Spinach Filling on page 79.

2	cups diced onions
1¼	cups diced bell peppers
1¾	cups diced mushrooms
2	cloves garlic, minced
	dash of black pepper
¼	teaspoon oregano
¼	teaspoon basil
1	cup cooked white rice
⅓	cup low-fat (1%) cottage cheese
2	tablespoons grated parmesan
3	tablespoons tomato paste
3	bell peppers, cut in half

Sauté the onions, peppers, mushrooms, and garlic in a little water, then mix in all the spices, rice, cottage cheese, parmesan, and tomato paste. Stuff the peppers and put them in a baking dish sprayed lightly with a nonstick spray. Bake in a preheated 350°F. oven for 1 hour, or until the peppers are soft.

Yield: 6 half-pepper servings

Calories per serving: 110
Fat: 1.1 g.
Sodium: 151 mg.

Creamed Onions with Sage

1	tablespoon margarine
5	teaspoons flour
1	cup chicken stock
1½	pounds pearl onions, peeled
¼	teaspoon black pepper
5	sage leaves, chopped
2	teaspoons low-fat plain yogurt
1	teaspoon chopped parsley

Make a roux by melting the margarine in a heavy saucepan and adding the flour, stirring constantly until a smooth paste forms and turns light brown. Gradually add the chicken stock, stirring to avoid lumps. Add the onions, and stir to lightly coat with sauce. Cover and cook over medium heat for 10 to 12 minutes, until the onions are soft and translucent. Add the pepper, chopped sage, yogurt, and parsley.

Yield: 6 ½-cup servings

Calories per serving: 70
Fat: 2.1 g.
Sodium: 27 mg.

Baked Tomatoes

4   fresh tomatoes
1   cup bread crumbs
4   cloves garlic, finely chopped
2   tablespoons chopped parsley
1   teaspoon ground thyme
1   teaspoon olive oil (optional)

The tomatoes do not have to be fully ripe. Cut the tomatoes in half. Do not peel them. Put the tomato halves on a baking sheet cut side up. Mix together the bread crumbs, garlic, parsley, and thyme. Sprinkle each tomato half with the mixture.

Drizzle each tomato half with the olive oil. (You may omit the olive oil, if desired.) Bake in a preheated 400°F. oven for 45 minutes.

Yield: 4 servings

Calories per serving: 140
Fat: 2.8 g.
Sodium: 196 mg.

Roasted Vegetables

2   pounds vegetables, such as summer
squash, zucchini, eggplant, carrots,
onions, tomatoes
cooking spray
seasonings

Wash the vegetables and cut into wedges. Place on a baking sheet lightly sprayed with cooking spray. Spray the vegetables with cooking spray. Season with your favorite spices; check the seasoning chart in Chapter 5 for some suggestions. Roast in a pre-heated 350°F. oven for 20 minutes or until the vegetables are soft and lightly browned.

Yield: 8–10 ½-cup servings

Calories per serving (est.): 30
Fat (est.): 1 g.
Sodium (est.): 15 mg.

Dijon Carrots and Zucchini

1½	cups carrots, cut into thin 2-inch sticks
2	tablespoons fat-free chicken broth
1½	cups zucchini, cut into thin 2-inch sticks
1	teaspoon apple cider vinegar
1	teaspoon honey
1½	teaspoons Dijon mustard

Combine the carrots and chicken broth in a saucepan. Cover and cook over medium heat for 10 minutes. Add the zucchini and cook an additional 5 minutes or until the vegetables are just tender. Add more broth, if necessary, to keep from burning. Stir the vinegar, honey, and mustard into the vegetables. Cook for a few minutes over medium heat until the liquid cooks off.

Yield: 6 ½-cup servings

Calories per serving: 27
Fat: .2 g.
Sodium: 43.1 mg.

Starches

Spanish Rice

1	tablespoon olive oil
2	cloves garlic, chopped
¾	teaspoon chili powder
1	cup white rice
¾	cup chopped green bell pepper
2	cups water
¼	teaspoon marjoram
1	16-ounce can low-salt whole tomatoes
½	teaspoon salt
1½	cups chopped onions

Heat the oil in a saucepan. Add the garlic, chili powder, and rice, and stir to coat the rice. Add the remaining ingredients and bring to a boil. Remove from the heat, cover with a lid or aluminum foil, and bake in a preheated 350°F. oven for 25 minutes.

Yield: 12 ⅓-cup servings

Calories per serving: 85
Fat: 1.4 g.
Sodium: 97 mg.

Kidney Beans and Rice

       2   cups dry red kidney beans
       1   cup chopped onions
       ½   cup diced green pepper
       ½   cup diced zucchini
       1   teaspoon canola oil
       2   cups cooked white rice

Cover beans with water and soak overnight. Drain, place in a pot with 6 cups of water, and cook for 1½ hours, adding water as necessary. Sauté the onions, pepper, and zucchini in the oil in a skillet. Add the beans and serve over the rice.

Yield: 4 servings
(Serving size: ¾ cup beans over ½ cup rice)

Calories per serving: 285
Fat: 3.1 g.
Sodium: 5.8 mg.

Roasted New Potatoes

2   pounds new potatoes
    cooking spray
2   teaspoons olive oil
1   teaspoon black pepper

Wash the potatoes and cut into wedges. Steam for 8 minutes, drain, and place on a baking sheet lightly sprayed with cooking spray. Drizzle the olive oil and black pepper over the potatoes. Roast in a pre-heated 450°F. oven for approximately 20 minutes, until browned.

Yield: 6 ½-cup servings

Calories per serving: 180
Fat: 1.7 g.
Sodium: 12 mg.

Mashed Potatoes

3½   pounds potatoes, peeled and diced
¾   cup buttermilk
¾   teaspoon salt

In a saucepan cover the potatoes with water and cook until soft. Drain; keep some of the liquid. Mash the potatoes; add the buttermilk, salt, and enough liquid until the potatoes have the right consistency.

This keeps well in the refrigerator for a few days.

Yield: 12 ½-cup servings

Calories per serving: 112
Fat: 0.3 g.
Sodium: 121 mg.

Sauces and
Stuffings

Fruit Stuffing

2	onions, diced
½	pound mushrooms, sliced
4	stalks celery, diced
1	teaspoon peanut oil
1	apple, peeled and diced
¼	cup dried apricots
1	cup chicken stock
5	cups bread cubes
2	teaspoons sage
¼	cup pecans
1	tablespoon thyme
½	teaspoon black pepper

Preheat the oven to 325°F. In a heavy pot sauté the onions, mushrooms, and celery in the oil until the onions are translucent. Add the apple and apricots. Cook for a few minutes and add the chicken stock. Bring to a boil, then remove from the heat. Toss the stock mixture with the remaining ingredients; place in a 10 × 10-inch baking pan sprayed with a non-stick cooking spray. Cover and bake for 30 minutes. Remove the cover and bake for 10 minutes more at 350°F.

Yield: 16 ½-cup servings   Calories per serving: 63
Fat: 2 g.
Sodium: 63 mg.

Vinaigrette

1   cup vegetable stock or water
1   tablespoon cornstarch
1   teaspoon mustard
1   clove garlic, minced
1   teaspoon salt
½   cup red wine vinegar
½   teaspoon black pepper
¼   cup olive oil

Boil the stock or water, remove from the heat, and add the cornstarch and dissolve in the heated liquid. Return to low heat and simmer, stirring to prevent lumps until it thickens. Combine the remaining ingredients and add to the thickened liquid. Cool and serve.

Yield: 16 2-tablespoon servings

Calories per serving: 14
Fat: 1.2 g.
Sodium: 120 mg.

Mock Sour Cream

1   cup low-fat cottage cheese
2   tablespoons skim milk
1   tablespoon lemon juice

In a blender mix the cottage cheese, skim milk, and lemon juice at high speed until smooth.

Yield: 1 cup

Calories, for 2 tablespoons: 22
Fat: 0.3 g.
Sodium: 117 mg.

Tartar Sauce

¼ cup chopped parsley
¾ cup fat-free mayonnaise
½ hard-boiled egg, chopped
2 tablespoons Dijon mustard
2 tablespoons lemon juice
1 tablespoon capers
2 tablespoons chopped scallions
1 tablespoon horseradish

Mix all the ingredients together and serve with the Salmon Cakes (page 91), if desired.

Yield: 12 2-tablespoon servings

Calories, for 2 tablespoons: 35
Fat: 2 g.
Sodium: 123 mg.

Lemon Mustard Dressing or Marinade

1   cup water
1   tablespoon cornstarch
4   tablespoons lemon juice
2   tablespoons chopped chives
2   tablespoons rice wine vinegar
4   tablespoons grainy Dijon mustard
1   tablespoon corn oil
2   tablespoons thinly sliced scallions

Bring the water to a boil; remove from the heat. Stir in the cornstarch until blended. Cool. Add the remaining ingredients and mix well.

Yield: 16 2-tablespoon servings

Calories, for 2 tablespoons: 12
Fat: 0.8 g.
Sodium: 40 mg.

Hummus

2	cups garbanzo beans, cooked
2	cloves garlic
2	tablespoons fresh lemon juice
¼	cup tahini (sesame butter)
¼	cup water
2	tablespoons chopped fresh parsley

Puree the ingredients, except the parsley, in a food processor or blender until smooth. Add the parsley and mix until just incorporated. Serve cold or at room temperature. Use as a dip or spread.

Yield: 12 ¼-cup servings

Calories per serving: 77
Fat: 3.5 g.
Sodium: 4 mg.

Creole Sauce

3   cups julienned or medium-diced
    onions
6   stalks celery, sliced ¼ inch on a slant
6   cloves garlic, minced or sliced
2   tablespoons peanut or canola oil
3   cups julienned or medium-diced
    green peppers
1   64-ounce can "no salt" tomatoes
2   tablespoons paprika
¼   cup Worcestershire sauce
½   teaspoon Tabasco

In a skillet sauté briefly the onions, celery, and garlic in the oil. Add the peppers, tomatoes, paprika,
Worcestershire, and Tabasco. Simmer on lowest
heat for 3 hours, stirring occasionally (it will reduce
by 50 percent). Serve with chicken or shrimp.

Yield: 12 ½-cup servings

Sauce:
Calories per serving: 80.5
Fat: 3 g.
Sodium: 39.4 mg.

Sauce with 5 shrimp per
  serving:
Calories: 151
Fat: 3.7 g.
Sodium: 199 mg.

Basil Sauce

1	clove garlic, minced
	pinch of salt
1	teaspoon mustard
1	tablespoon mayonnaise
½	cup low-fat yogurt
¼	cup chopped basil
1	tablespoon chopped parsley

Combine all the ingredients, mix well, and store in the refrigerator. You can serve this as a spread for sandwiches.

Yield: 12 1-tablespoon servings

Calories per serving: 21
Fat: 1.5 g.
Sodium: 54 mg.

Salads and
Soups

Lentil Salad

½	pound lentils
½	cup diced red onions
1	clove garlic, minced
¼	cup chopped parsley
1	tablespoon lemon juice
1	teaspoon black pepper
½	cup diced carrots
½	cup low-fat yogurt
1	cup seeded and diced tomatoes
½	cup Vinaigrette (page 114)
1	teaspoon ground cumin
1	teaspoon salt

Cook the lentils in two to three quarts of water until soft but not mushy. Combine the remaining ingredients with the cooked lentils. Cool and serve.

Yield: 15 ⅓-cup servings

Calories per serving: 69
Fat: 0.7 g.
Sodium: 185 mg.

Sesame Noodle Salad

1	pound spaghetti
4	cloves garlic
1	1-inch piece ginger
½	cup tahini
1½	teaspoons brown sugar
¼	cup soy sauce
2	tablespoons peanut oil
¼	cup sherry vinegar
½	cup water
½	pound yellow squash
½	pound zucchini
¼	pound snow peas
1	medium red pepper
½	cup scallions
	parsley or coriander leaves, chopped

Cook the spaghetti al dente; rinse and set aside. In a food processor mince the garlic and ginger, add the tahini and brown sugar, and process until smooth. Slowly add the soy sauce, peanut oil, and vinegar. Add water as needed. Julienne all the vegetables and add to the salad. Garnish with chopped parsley or coriander leaves.

Yield: 9 4-ounce servings   Calories per serving: 146
Fat: 5.7 g.
Sodium: 233 mg.

Carrot Salad

6	cups grated carrots
6	tablespoons lemon juice
½	cup chopped parsley
1½	tablespoons mustard
½	teaspoon salt
½	teaspoon black pepper

Combine the carrots with all the remaining ingredients. Mix well. Let stand for 1 hour before serving.

Yield: 8 4-ounce servings

Calories per serving: 40.5
Fat: .35 g.
Sodium: 160 mg.

Garden Peas Salad

1   package (16 ounces) frozen peas
½   cup nonfat plain yogurt
2   teaspoons reduced-calorie mayonnaise
½   cup chopped onions or scallions
½   teaspoon dried dill (if using fresh, can
     add more)

Cook the peas following the package instructions. Drain and let cool. To make the dressing, in a small bowl mix together the yogurt, mayonnaise, onions, and dill. Toss this mixture with the peas. Cover and refrigerate until ready to serve.

Yield: 4 ½-cup servings

Calories per serving: 118
Fat: 2 g.
Sodium: 160 mg.

Basil Chicken Salad

1¼	pounds skinless, boneless chicken breast
½	cup dried barley
4	cups water
½	cup diced celery
½	cup diced onion
¼	cup diced apples
¼	cup nonfat plain yogurt
½	tablespoon salt
2	tablespoons chopped parsley
¼	cup chopped fresh basil
2	tablespoons mayonnaise (light or nonfat)
1	clove garlic, minced
¼	cup buttermilk
	juice of 1 lemon and grated rind of 1 lemon
¼	teaspoon black pepper

Poach or steam the chicken and let cool. Trim and cut into 1-inch cubes. Meanwhile cook the barley in the water; let cool. Combine the chicken and barley with all the remaining ingredients and serve.

Yield: 15 ⅔-cup servings

Calories per serving: 171
Fat: 4.5 g.
Sodium: 243 mg.

Turkey Corn Salad

1	pound cooked turkey breast
1½	pounds frozen corn
2	cups tomatoes, seeded and diced
½	cup coarsely chopped fresh coriander leaves
½	cup Vinaigrette (page 114)

Trim the turkey and cut into ½-inch cubes. Cook the corn according to package directions, cool, and add to the turkey along with the tomatoes and coriander. Prepare Vinaigrette. Add ½ cup Vinaigrette to the salad, toss, and serve. Garnish with the fresh coriander leaves.

Yield: 9 6-ounce servings

Calories per serving: 182
Fat: 2.78 g.
Sodium: 110 mg.

Tomato Bisque

3½	cups chopped onions
½	cup chopped celery
½	cup chopped carrots
¾	tablespoon olive oil
1	teaspoon tarragon
¼	teaspoon thyme
¼	cup raw rice
3	pounds tomatoes, seeded and chopped
5	cups chicken or vegetable stock
½	cup tomato paste
1	bay leaf
½	cup chopped fresh basil
¼	teaspoon salt
¼	teaspoon black pepper

Sauté the vegetables in the oil and add the tarragon and thyme. Add the rice, tomatoes, and stock. Bring to a boil; add the tomato paste and the bay leaf. Simmer for 30 minutes, until the vegetables are al dente. Add the basil, salt, and black pepper and puree. Reheat and serve.

Yield: 10 1-cup servings

Calories per serving: 64
Fat: 0.9 g.
Sodium: 164 mg.

White Bean Soup

½   pound white beans
12   cups water
½   teaspoon salt
     dash of pepper
     pinch of ground cloves
1   bay leaf
1   cup onions, diced very small
1   cup celery, diced very small
2   carrots, diced very small
2   tablespoons chopped fresh parsley
1   16-ounce can whole plum tomatoes

Cook the beans in the water, with the salt, pepper, cloves, and bay leaf for 2 to 3 hours. When the beans are soft, discard the bay leaf, add the remaining ingredients, and simmer until the vegetables are soft, about 30 minutes. Add vegetable stock or water as needed.

Yield: 9 1-cup servings

Calories per serving: 114
Fat: 0.6 g.
Sodium: 150 mg.

Split Pea Soup

3	cups diced onions
1½	cups diced carrots
1½	cups diced celery
	cooking spray
1	bay leaf
½	teaspoon thyme
1	teaspoon salt
½	teaspoon black pepper
1	pound split peas, cleaned
9	cups water

In a skillet, sauté the onions, carrots, and celery in cooking spray. Cook until the onions are transparent. Add the herbs, spices, peas, and water. Bring to a boil, skim, then simmer partially covered for 2½ to 3 hours, or until thick.

Yield: 12 1-cup servings

Calories per serving: 153
Fat: 5 g.
Sodium: 163 mg.

Breads, Cakes, and Desserts

Blueberry Pancakes

1½	cups flour or 1 cup white flour and ½ cup whole wheat flour
2	tablespoons sugar
1	teaspoon baking powder
½	teaspoon baking soda
1½	cups buttermilk
1	egg
1	cup blueberries
2	tablespoons water

Separately mix the dry and wet ingredients, except the blueberries. Combine the dry and wet ingredients, leaving the mixture somewhat lumpy. Stir in the blueberries or add to each pancake while cooking. Cook in a nonstick skillet for 2 minutes on each side. Serve immediately.

Yield: 10 pancakes (2 ounces batter per pancake)

Calories per serving: 104
Fat: 1g.
Sodium: 120 mg.

Apple Cake

4   medium apples, peeled
2   eggs
1   tablespoon vanilla extract
1   cup sugar
1   cup white flour
2   teaspoons cinnamon
2   teaspoons baking powder

Dice the apples; combine with the eggs, beaten with the vanilla and sugar. Combine the flour, cinnamon, and baking powder. Mix all the ingredients and bake in a 9 × 9-inch baking pan in a preheated 350°F. oven for 15 to 20 minutes.

Yield: 16 servings

Calories per serving: 105
Fat: 0.8 g.
Sodium: 49 mg.

Apple Crisp

6	cups sliced apples
¾	cup apple juice
1	cup crumbled cinnamon graham crackers
1½	teaspoons nutmeg
1	tablespoon reduced-calorie margarine, melted

Grease a 9 × 13-inch pan with nonstick spray. Layer the apples in the pan. Pour the apple juice over the apples. Mix the remaining ingredients and sprinkle over the apple mixture. Bake, covered, for 20 minutes in a preheated 350°F. oven, or until the apples are soft. Uncover and bake 20 minutes more.

Yield: 8 servings

Calories per serving: 80
Fat: 1 g.
Sodium: 34 mg.

Blueberry Cake

⅔ cup applesauce
1 cup sugar
2 eggs
1 cup nonfat vanilla yogurt
½ teaspoon baking soda
1 tablespoon baking powder
1 teaspoon nutmeg
2 cups flour
2 cups blueberries

In separate bowls combine the dry ingredients and the wet ingredients, except the blueberries. Mix the dry and wet ingredients together, adding the blueberries when the mixture is just blended. Spray a 9 × 9-inch pan with cooking spray and pour in the batter. Bake in a preheated 350°F. oven for 50 minutes.

Yield: 16 pieces

Calories per piece: 148
Fat: 1.1 g.
Sodium: 107 mg.

Corn Bread

1½	cups cornmeal
½	cup all-purpose flour
1	tablespoon baking powder
½	teaspoon baking soda
2	tablespoons apple juice concentrate
1⅓	cups buttermilk
2	egg whites

Preheat the oven to 400°F. Spray an 8 × 8-inch pan with nonstick spray. Mix the dry ingredients and set aside. Mix the apple juice and buttermilk. In a mixer beat the egg whites until stiff. Add the cornmeal mixture to the buttermilk and mix with a fork. Fold in the egg whites. Bake immediately in the oven for 20 minutes, or until browned.

Yield: 12 2 × 2-inch servings

Calories per serving: 93
Fat: 0.8 g.
Sodium: 160 mg.

Sponge Cake with Fresh Fruit

3	egg yolks
3	tablespoons water
2	tablespoons lemon juice
1	teaspoon lemon zest
1	cup sugar
¾	cup cake flour, plus extra for dusting
¼	teaspoon salt
6	egg whites
	sliced fresh fruit

Beat the egg yolks with the water, lemon juice, lemon zest, and sugar. Fold in the flour and salt. Beat the egg whites into stiff peaks and fold into the flour mixture. Spray a 9 × 9-inch pan with nonstick cooking spray and dust with flour. Pour in the batter and bake for 30 minutes in a preheated 350°F. oven. Cool before cutting. Serve with sliced fresh fruit.

Yield: 12 servings

Calories per serving: 125 (plus fruit)
Fat: 1.6 g.
Sodium: 78 mg.

Molasses Cookies

1½	cups flour
2½	cups dry oatmeal
1⅙	cups oat bran
2	teaspoons cinnamon
¾	teaspoon dry ginger
1½	teaspoons baking soda
¼	teaspoon salt
⅛	teaspoon cloves
5	egg whites
1	cup sugar
⅓	cup molasses
⅛	cup apple juice
½	cup oil
1	cup sugar (for rolling the cookies)

Mix together the flour, oatmeal, oat bran, cinnamon, ginger, baking soda, salt, and cloves, using a hand mixer. Mix together the egg whites, 1 cup sugar, molasses, juice, and oil. Combine the wet and dry ingredients together on low speed until moist. Refrigerate the batter for 1 hour. Use a 2-ounce scoop to measure the cookies. Shape a cookie into a ball, roll it in sugar, then press down with a rolling pin (or jar) on a greased sheet pan. Bake the cookies in a preheated 350°F. oven for 8 minutes.

Yield: 36 cookies

Calories per cookie: 95.7
Fat: 3.2 g.
Sodium: 58 mg.

Gingerbread

½ cup molasses
1 cup buttermilk
2 tablespoons peanut oil
6 egg whites
½ teaspoon baking powder
2 cups all-purpose flour
⅔ cup brown sugar
2 teaspoons ground ginger
1 teaspoon baking soda
½ teaspoon nutmeg
½ teaspoon allspice

Combine all the wet ingredients in one bowl and all the dry ingredients in another. Pour the wet ingredient mixture over the dry mixture and fold in gently. Pour into a 10 × 10-inch pan sprayed with nonstick cooking spray. Bake in a preheated 350°F. oven for 25 minutes.

Yield: 20 servings

Calories per serving: 113
Fat: 1.6 g.
Sodium: 90 mg.

Raspberry Streusel Bars

1	cup bran cereal
¾	cup all-purpose flour
¾	cup whole wheat flour
½	cup firmly packed brown sugar
½	teaspoon baking soda
¼	teaspoon cinnamon
¼	cup reduced-calorie margarine
¼	cup water
½	cup raspberry fruit spread

In a medium mixing bowl, combine the bran cereal, flours, brown sugar, baking soda, and cinnamon. Using a pastry blender or two knives, cut in the margarine until the mixture resembles coarse crumbs. Stir in the water; the mixture should be crumbly. Set aside 1 cup of the mixture. With the back of a spoon, press the remaining mixture firmly into the bottom of an 8 × 8 × 2-inch baking pan sprayed with nonstick cooking spray. Spread the raspberry fruit spread evenly over the cereal mixture in the bottom of the pan. Sprinkle with the reserved cereal mixture. Bake in a preheated 350°F. oven for about

25 minutes, or until lightly browned. Cool before serving.

Yield: 16 bars

Calories per bar: 101
Fat: 2 g.
Sodium: 104 mg.

Lemon Muffins

3	tablespoons margarine
1	egg
1	tablespoon fresh lemon juice
1	tablespoon lemon zest
¼	teaspoon lemon extract
1¾	cups all-purpose flour
¾	cup sugar
1	teaspoon baking soda
¼	teaspoon salt
1	cup nonfat plain yogurt

In separate bowls combine the wet and the dry ingredients. Mix the wet and dry ingredients together until just blended. Spray a muffin pan with cooking spray. Bake in a preheated 350°F. oven for about 12 minutes.

Yield: 12 muffins

Calories per muffin: 159
Fat: 3.7 g.
Sodium: 176 mg.

Blueberry Muffins

⅔	cup all-purpose flour
⅔	cup whole wheat flour
2¾	teaspoons baking powder
¾	teaspoon baking soda
2	teaspoons cinnamon
⅓	cup oatmeal
⅓	cup oat bran
⅔	cup wheat germ
⅓	cup sugar
⅓	cup raisins
1	banana
1	cup blueberries
5	egg whites, beaten
1	tablespoon plus 1 teaspoon canola oil
⅓	cup skim milk
1	tablespoon plus 1 teaspoon orange juice

In separate bowls combine the dry ingredients and the wet ingredients. Mix the wet and dry ingredients together until just blended. Do not over-mix. Spray a muffin pan with cooking spray. Bake in a preheated 350°F. oven for 25 minutes. Cool before serving.

Yield: 12 muffins

Calories per muffin: 153
Fat: 2.6 g.
Sodium: 166 mg.

Resources and
Further Reading

Additional information and advice can be obtained from the following sources:

American Dietetic Association: 1-800-877-1600

Citizens for Public Action on Blood Pressure and Cholesterol, P.O. Box 30374, Bethesda, MD 20824, 301-770-1711

Learning to Live with Hypertension, published in 1983 by Medicine in the Public Interest, Suite 400, One State St., Boston, MA 02109

National Heart, Lung, and Blood Institute Information Center, P.O. Box 30105, Bethesda, MD 20824-0105, 301-251-1222

NHLBI Blood Pressure Hot Line: 1-800-575-WELL

Index

Italic entries refer to recipes.

adrenal glands, 26
African Americans, 18, 25
alcohol, 4, 5, 6, 7, 17, 20–22, 47
  calories from, 21, 45, 47
  recommended daily amount
    of, 21–22, 47
angina, 14–15
antihypertensive drugs, *see*
  medication, hypertension
apple(s), 40, 42
  Cake, 133
  Crisp, 134
apricots, 36, 40, 50
arteries, 9–10, 20, 31
  hardening of (arterio-
    sclerosis), 10, 14–15, 21
  potassium and, 26
  see also heart disease
arterioles, 9–10
  strokes and, 15–16
arteriosclerosis (hardening of the
  arteries), 10, 14–15, 21
asparagus, seasonings for, 52

bananas, 36, 42
Basil:
  Chicken Salad, 126
  Sauce, 120

bass, 29
bean(s), 26, 36, 40, 44, 46
  Beef Chili, 98
  green, 36, 53
  Hummus, 118
  Kidney, and Rice, 109
  magnesium in, 37
  Moroccan Vegetable Stew,
    81–82
  White, Soup, 129
beef, 29
  Chili, 98
  fat in, 44, 51–52
  Marinated Flank Steak, 99
  potassium in, 37
  seasonings for, 53
  sodium in, 37
black-eyed peas, 36, 38
blood clots, 29
blood pressure, 9–10
  high, *see* hypertension
  measurement of, 11–13
blood pressure medication, *see*
  medication, hypertension
Blueberry:
  Cake, 135
  Muffins, 143
  Pancakes, 132

bluefish, 29
body weight, *see* weight
breads, 7, 32, 40, 46, 50, 51, 65
 Blueberry Muffins, 143
 Blueberry Pancakes, 132
 Corn, 136
 Fruit Stuffing, 113
 Lemon Muffins, 142
broccoli, 36, 38, 40, 42
 seasonings for, 53
butter, 46, 49
buying food, 48–52

cabbage, 42
cakes, 47, 51
 Apple, 133
 Blueberry, 135
 Gingerbread, 139
 Sponge, with Fresh Fruit,
 137
calcium, 4, 6, 7, 17, 18, 23, 27,
 28, 38
 recommended daily amount
 of, 38
 sources of, 38, 42, 52
 supplemental, 28
calories, 44–45, 46, 47
 from alcohol, 21, 45, 47
 from complex carbohydrates,
 40, 44
 from fat, 44, 45, 46–47
 in McDonald's lunches, 61
 nutrition label information
 on, 56
 weight control and, 72–73
cantaloupes, 42
carbohydrates, complex
 (starches), 33, 40–41, 48, 51,
 65
 calories from, 40, 44
 Kidney Beans and Rice, 109
 Mashed Potatoes, 111
 recommended daily amount
 of, 41
 Roasted New Potatoes, 110
 sources of, 40
 Spanish Rice, 108
cardiovascular disease, *see*
 arteries; heart disease

Carrot(s):
 Salad, 124
 and Zucchini, Dijon, 106
Catfish, Baked, 89
cauliflower, 42
cereals, 32, 40, 46
cheese, 26, 38, 46, 52, 77
chicken, 29, 46, 62
 Grilled, 86
 with Saffron Rice, 84–85
 Salad, Basil, 126
 Stir-Fry, 83
Chili, Beef, 98
Chinese food, 63
cholesterol, 46
 exercise and, 20
 HDL, 21
cookies, 47, 51
 Molasses, 138
 Raspberry Streusel Bars,
 140–41
cooking, 49, 58–59
 seasonings in, 35, 52–54, 59
 substituting ingredients in, 77
 of vegetables, 42, 52–54
corn:
 seasonings for, 53
 Turkey Salad, 127
Corn Bread, 136
coronary disease, *see* arteries;
 heart disease
cream, 46

daily value, on nutrition labels,
 56
dairy products, 7, 32, 50, 65
 calcium in, 38, 42, 52
 cheese, 26, 38, 46, 52, 77
 magnesium in, 37
 milk, 26, 37, 38, 42, 43, 52, 77
 potassium in, 37, 52
 sodium in, 37
 yogurt, 37, 38, 47, 77
dates, 36
deli foods, 64
desserts, 43, 47, 49, 51
 Apple Cake, 133
 Apple Crisp, 134
 Blueberry Cake, 135

Gingerbread, 139
Molasses Cookies, 138
Raspberry Streusel Bars,
    140–41
Sponge Cake with Fresh Fruit,
    137
dialysis, 17
diuretics, 39
diets, 69
    vegetarian, 4, 6, 49
    see also nutrition, nutrients;
        weight control
dressings, *see* salad dressings
drugs, hypertension, *see*
    medication, hypertension

eating out, 60–66
    at fast food restaurants, 61–63
eggs, 43, 46
    seasonings for, 53
exercise, 20, 21, 69
    in weight control, 75–76
eye damage, 16

fast food restaurants, 61–63
fat-free products, 46
    dairy, 37, 38, 52, 77
fats, 4, 6, 7, 19, 33, 40, 41, 44–47,
    48, 49, 51, 52, 65
    calories from, 44, 45, 46–47
    exercise and, 20
    in fast foods, 61, 62, 63, 64
    food diary and, 73
    in meats, 44, 51–52
    nutrition label information
        on, 56
    recommended daily amount
        of, 45, 46
    saturated, 46, 51–52
    see also cholesterol
fiber, 30, 39
    nutrition label information
        on, 56
    recommended daily amount
        of, 39
    sources of, 39, 40, 41, 42
fish and shellfish, 38, 44, 51
    Baked Catfish, 89
    Baked Grouper, 93

in fast food restaurants, 62
Flounder Stuffed with
    Mushrooms, 94
omega-3 oils in, 28–29, 44,
    51
potassium in, 37
Salmon Cakes, 91–92
seasonings for, 53
Sesame Mahimahi, 90
Shrimp Scampi, 95–96
sodium in, 37
Flounder Stuffed with
    Mushrooms, 94
food diary, 73–74
food pyramid, 32, 40, 50, 65
    pictured, 32
French fries, 61, 62
fried foods, 49, 62, 63, 64
frozen foods, 50, 52
fruit(s), 6, 7, 19, 32, 38, 40, 41,
    42–43, 45, 48, 65
    buying of, 50, 51
    fiber in, 39, 41
    Fresh, Sponge Cake with, 137
    frozen, 50
    meals of, 43
    potassium in, 26, 36, 41, 42
    recommended daily amount
        of, 41
    sodium in, 36, 41
    Stuffing, 113

genetic susceptibility to risk
    factors, 17
Gingerbread, 139
grains, 7, 19, 28, 32, 40, 51
    breads, *see* breads
    cereals, 32, 40, 46
    fiber in, 39
    magnesium in, 28, 37
    pasta, *see* pasta
    rice, *see* rice
grapes, 42
green beans,   36, 53
Grouper, Baked, 93

halibut, 29
heart, 9
heart attacks, 15, 20, 29, 45

heart disease, 1, 2, 6, 11, 14–15, 31
  heart attacks, 15, 20, 29, 45
  omega-3 oils and, 29, 51
  see also arteries
herbs and spices, 35, 52–54, 59
heredity, 17
herring, 29
Honey-Mustard Tenderloin, 100
hot dogs, 62
Hummus, 118
hunger, 74
hypertension (high blood pressure), 1–2, 10–11
  effects of, 1–2, 15–17; *see also specific conditions*
  medication for, *see* medication, hypertension
  risk factors for, 17–22; *see also specific risk factors*
  stages of, 11, 13
  white coat, 13

inactivity, 20, 31, 75
  see also exercise
Indian food, 64
Intersalt, 4–5
ischemia, 15

Japanese food, 63

kale, 38
kidney disease, 2, 11, 16–17
kidneys:
  potassium and, 26
  sodium and, 17–18, 24, 25

labels, nutrition, 54–58
lamb, seasonings for, 53
left ventricular hypertrophy, 14
legumes, 28
  black-eyed peas, 36, 38
  lentils, 36
  Lentil Salad, 122
  potassium in, 36
  sodium in, 36
  see also bean
Lemon:
  Muffins, 142

Mustard Dressing or Marinade, 117
lentil(s), 36
  Salad, 122
lettuce, 40, 42

McDonald's restaurants, 61
mackerel, 29
magnesium, 18, 23, 27–28
  recommended daily amount of, 37
  sources of, 28, 37–38
  supplemental, 27–28
Mahimahi, Sesame, 90
main dishes:
  Baked Catfish, 89
  Baked Grouper, 93
  Beef Chili, 98
  Chicken Stir-Fry, 83
  Chicken with Saffron Rice, 84–85
  Flounder Stuffed with Mushrooms, 94
  Grilled Chicken, 86
  Honey-Mustard Tenderloin, 100
  Marinated Flank Steak, 99
  Moroccan Vegetable Stew, 81–82
  Pearl Balls, 88
  Roast Turkey Breast, 87
  Salmon Cakes, 91–92
  Sesame Mahimahi, 90
  Shrimp and Green Peas, 97
  Shrimp Scampi, 95–96
  Spinach-Stuffed Shells, 79–80
margarine, 49
Marinade, Lemon Mustard, 117
meats, 7, 32, 43, 46, 50, 65
  beef, *see* beef
  daily servings of, 43–44, 51
  deli, 64
  fat in, 44, 51–52
  lamb, 53
  pork, *see* pork
  potassium in, 37
  seasonings for, 53, 54
  sodium in, 37
  veal, 54

medication, hypertension, 2–4,
22
  alcohol and, 21
  diuretics, 39
  potassium and, 26
Mexican food, 63
Middle Eastern food, 64
milk, 26, 37, 38, 42, 43, 52, 77
Molasses:
  Cookies, 138
  Gingerbread, 139
muffins, 51
  Blueberry, 143
  Lemon, 142
mushrooms, 36
  Flounder Stuffed with, 94
mustard, 49
  *Dijon Carrots and Zucchini,
  106*
  Honey Tenderloin, 100
  *Lemon Dressing or Marinade,
  117*
myocardial infarctions (heart
  attacks), 15, 20, 29

National Institutes of Health
  (NIH), 10–11
  National High Blood Pressure
  Education Program of, 2
noodle:
  Salad, Sesame, 123
  see also pasta
nutrition, nutrients, 3–8, 19–20,
  22, 23–30, 31–47
  alcohol, see alcohol
  calcium, see calcium
  carbohydrates, see
  carbohydrates, complex
  fats, see fats
  fiber, see fiber
  food labels and, 54–58
  food pyramid and, 32, 40, 50,
  65
  fruit, see fruit
  magnesium, see magnesium
  omega-3 fatty acids, 28–29, 44,
  51
  potassium, see potassium
  protein, 43, 44

sodium, see salt and sodium
  sugars, 7, 40, 47, 65
  supplemental, 27–28, 38–39
  vegetables, see vegetable
nuts, 26, 37

obesity and overweight, 4, 6,
  19–20, 41, 68
  waist-to-hip ratio and, 19,
  71–72
  see also weight control
oils, 46, 49
  see also fats
omega-3 fatty acids, 28–29, 44,
  51
Onions, Creamed, with Sage, 103
orange juice, 36
oranges, 42

Pancakes, Blueberry, 132
pasta, 40, 46, 50, 51
  Sesame Noodle Salad, 123
  Shrimp Scampi, 95–96
  Spinach-Stuffed Shells, 79–80
pea(s), 40
  Garden, Salad, 125
  Green, Shrimp and, 97
  seasonings for, 53
  Split, Soup, 130
Pearl Balls, 88
Peppers, Stuffed, 102
pickles, 64
pies, 51
pork, 29, 44
  *Honey-Mustard Tenderloin,
  100*
  seasonings for, 53
potassium, 4, 5, 6, 7, 18, 21,
  23–24, 25, 26, 28, 39
  genetic sensitivities and, 17
  increasing intake of, 35–36,
  50
  recommended daily amount
  of, 36
  sodium and, 18, 23–24, 25, 26,
  27
  sources of, 26, 28, 36–37,
  41–42, 52
  supplemental, 39

potato chips, 33, 34, 45, 48–49, 66–67
potatoes, 26, 36, 40, 62
   Mashed, 111
   Roasted New, 110
   seasonings for, 53–54
poultry, 43
   Pearl Balls, 88
   Roast Turkey Breast, 87
   seasonings for, 53
   Turkey Corn Salad, 127
   see also chicken
processed foods, 24, 26, 34, 35, 50, 58
   nutrition labels on, 54–58
protein, 43–44
   calories from, 44

Raspberry Streusel Bars, 140–41
recipes, substituting ingredients in, 77
renal disease (kidney disease), 2, 11, 16–17
restaurants, 60–66
   fast food, 61–63
retina, 16
rice, 40, 41, 51
   Kidney Beans and, 109
   Pearl Balls, 88
   Saffron, Chicken with, 84–85
   Spanish, 108

Saffron Rice, Chicken with, 84–85
Sage, Creamed Onions with, 103
salad dressings:
   Lemon Mustard, 117
   Vinaigrette, 114
salads, 42, 62, 64, 65
   Basil Chicken, 126
   Carrot, 124
   Garden Peas, 125
   Lentil, 122
   Sesame Noodle, 123
   Turkey Corn, 127
salmon, 29, 37
   Cakes, 91–92
salt and sodium, 4, 5–6, 23–25, 26, 41

   cutting intake of, 7, 21, 23, 25, 33–35, 39, 48–49, 50, 58–59
   exercise and, 20
   in fast food, 61, 62, 63, 64
   food diary and, 73
   foods low in, 36–37
   in frozen meals, 52
   hidden sources of, 34, 57, 58
   nutrition label information on, 57–58
   potassium and, 18, 23–24, 25, 26, 27
   recommended daily amount of, 24, 34
   sensitivity to, 17–18, 24–25, 27, 28
   sources of, 24, 26, 34–35, 48–49, 50, 52, 57–58, 61, 62, 63, 64
sardines, 29, 38
sauces:
   Basil, 120
   Creole, 119
   Hummus, 118
   Lemon Mustard Dressing or Marinade, 117
   Mock Sour Cream, 115
   Tartar, 116
   Vinaigrette, 114
scallops, 37
seasonings, 35, 52–54, 59
serving sizes, on nutrition labels, 54
Sesame:
   Mahimahi, 90
   Noodle Salad, 123
shark, 29
shortening, 46, 49
Shrimp:
   and Green Peas, 97
   Scampi, 95–96
silent ischemia, 15
snacks, 43, 48–49, 50, 64
   potato chips, 33, 34, 45, 48–49, 66–67
sodium, *see* salt and sodium
soups, 65, 77
   Split Pea, 130

Tomato Bisque, 128
White Bean, 129
sour cream, 77
  Mock, 115
spices and herbs, 35, 52–54, 59
spinach, 36, 38, 41
  Stuffed Shells, 79–80
squid, 29
starches, *see* carbohydrates,
    complex
Stew, Moroccan Vegetable, 81–82
Stir-Fry, Chicken, 83
stress, 17
strokes, 1, 2, 11, 15–16, 21, 31
  hemorrhagic, 21
  inactivity and, 20
  omega-3 oils and, 29
  potassium and, 26
  salt and, 26
Stuffing, Fruit, 113
sugar and sweets, 7, 40, 47, 65
  see also desserts

Tartar Sauce, 116
Thai food, 64
tomato(es), 36
  Baked, 104
  Bisque, 128
  seasonings for, 54
trout, 29, 37
tuna, 37
Turkey:
  Breast, Roast, 87
  Corn Salad, 127
  Pearl Balls, 88
turnip greens, 38

veal, seasonings for, 54
vegetable(s), 6, 7, 19, 32, 40,
    41–42, 46, 48, 65
  Baked Tomatoes, 104
  buying of, 50, 51
  calcium in, 38

cooking of, 42, 52–54
Creamed Onions with Sage,
  103
Dijon Carrots and Zucchini,
  106
fiber in, 39, 41, 42
frozen, 50, 52
magnesium in, 28, 37–38
Mashed Potatoes, 111
potassium in, 26, 28, 36, 41–42
recommended daily amount
  of, 41, 44
Roasted, 105
Roasted New Potatoes, 110
seasonings for, 52–54
sodium in, 36, 41
Stew, Moroccan, 81–82
Stuffed Peppers, 102
vegetarian diet, 4, 6, 49
Vinaigrette, 114
vinegar, 59
vitamins and supplements,
  27–28, 38–39

watermelon, 36, 42
weight, 5, 7, 17
  suggested, 70, 71
  see also obesity and overweight
weight control, 19, 21, 68–76
  calories and, 72–73
  emotional eating and, 74–75
  exercise and, 75–76
  food diary and, 73–74
  health assessment and, 70–71
  suggested weight and, 70, 71
  waist-to-hip ratio and, 71–72
whitefish, 29
wine, 21

yogurt, 37, 38, 47, 77

Zucchini and Carrots, Dijon, 106